Taking control

Bladder and bowel problems

Kerry Lee

**Published by
Age Concern England
1268 London Road
London SW16 4ER**

© 2005 Age Concern England

First published 2005

Editor Ro Lyon

Production Leonie Farmer

A catalogue record for this book is available
from the British Library.

ISBN-13: 978-0-86242-386-5
ISBN-10: 0-86242-386-4

While every effort has been made to check
the accuracy of material contained in this
publication, Age Concern England cannot
accept responsibility for the results of any
action taken by readers as a result of reading
this book. Please note that while the agen-
cies or products mentioned in this book are
known to Age Concern, inclusion here does
not constitute a recommendation by Age
Concern for any particular product, agency,
service or publication.

Design and typesetting: www.Intertype.com

Printed in Great Britain by Bell & Bain Ltd, Glasgow

Contents

About the author

Kerry Lee works as Communications Manager for *In*contact, a leading UK charity that supports people with bladder and bowel problems. Her role includes producing patient information leaflets and the magazine which is sent to all *In*contact members. In addition, Kerry helps to take calls to the office from people with bladder and bowel problems, and from healthcare professionals, who want to find out more about *In*contact and the work it does. Kerry is also the main point of contact for any PR-related enquiries.

Kerry lives in Hertfordshire with her partner and her two cats. She enjoys writing fiction and is currently completing an interior design diploma.

Acknowledgements

I would like to thank all those who helped with the research for this book, including *In*contact staff (past and present), the Medical Advisory Board and members of *In*contact's Publications Advisory Committee.

I also thank the *In*contact members who provide many of the case studies used throughout the book.

My thanks also go to Richard Holloway and all at Age Concern England for the help and support they have given me along the way.

Kerry Lee

Introduction

Many people have bladder and bowel problems. A telephone survey in 2002 (*Healthy Bladder Campaign* by SMS Ltd) found that 7 in 10 people in the UK have, or have had, a bladder problem at some time in their lives. The Continence Foundation estimates that 500,000 adults have bowel incontinence.

Bladder and bowel problems can affect both men and women, of all ages. The problems can range from urgency, frequency, or perhaps a slight leak, to total loss of bladder and bowel control. No two people will have exactly the same problem, but you are likely to experience some similar feelings: anxiety, embarrassment and despair.

This book will provide answers to your questions and help you feel more in control of your problem.

Bowel and bladder problems are still a taboo subject. People often think they are the only one with a problem and don't even tell their closest family and friends about it. Likewise, lots of people with bladder and bowel problems don't seek professional advice, or even know who to turn to for help. Organisations such as *In*contact are constantly trying to raise awareness of these problems and to ensure that people know who to contact for information about products and services.

It is important to remember, however, that bladder and bowel problems aren't just an inevitable part of ageing. Not every older person has a bladder or bowel problem (and younger people can have them too). But if you do have problems, many things can be done to help. You don't need to live with the problem and it is important to seek professional help – this book explains the roles of different health professionals and the possible treatments that they may offer you.

A bladder or bowel problem doesn't just affect you physically – it can affect your emotional well-being as well. You don't have to cope with your problem alone. There are organisations that can offer help and advice and put you in touch with others who 'know what it's like'.

There are also many ways to manage your problem. Products which can help you cope are improving all the time: a list of useful contacts is provided at the back of the book on pages 99–104.

Whatever your bladder or bowel problem, this book provides information, advice and tips from people with these conditions.

Chapter 1 outlines the causes of bladder and bowel problems. It covers long-term conditions and injuries, and the specific bladder and bowel problems that arise because of them.

Chapter 2 introduces the range of treatments and management options available to you. It also outlines the different roles of the healthcare professionals who can help, and how to communicate effectively with them.

Chapter 3 covers the related issues that can arise from having to deal with a bladder or bowel problem, such as emotional worry and stress and continuing with your sex life.

Chapter 4 provides in-depth information about the bladder: how it works; the types of bladder problems; and the treatment and management choices for people with those problems.

Chapter 5 provides comprehensive information about the bowel: how it works; the types of bowel problems; and the treatment and management choices for people with those problems.

The glossary on pages 93–98 explains what the technical terms mean.

You may have bladder or bowel problems, or you may be caring for someone with these problems. The problems may be slight, or may be more severe. Whoever you are, and whatever your problem, you are not alone.

Beatrice
'I'm 80 and used to think that bladder problems were an inevitable part of ageing. Now I realise that there are many things that can be done to help and bladder problems affect people of all ages.'

1 Causes of bladder and bowel problems

Just as there are many different types of bladder and bowel problems, so, too, are there many different causes. Whether you have been born with a problem, or have a problem as a result of an accident or disease, remember that you aren't the only one in this situation. Although no-one's condition is exactly the same as the next person's, bladder and bowel problems affect the lives of millions of people. Many factors can cause, or contribute to, bladder and bowel problems. These include diseases which affect the nervous system, mental health problems, and some operations and injuries. This chapter outlines the types of bladder and bowel problems that can arise. Details of how to help manage these problems appear later in the book.

Multiple sclerosis

Multiple sclerosis (MS) is a condition which affects the central nervous system. It is caused by damage to the protective covering of the nerve fibres. Signals from and to the brain are disrupted.

People with MS are likely to have bladder problems. The bladder is controlled by nerves from the spinal cord. If these nerves are damaged, then you may not know when your bladder needs emptying, or be able to send the right messages to the muscles that prevent urine leakage.

Many people with early symptoms of MS find that they have *frequency* (needing the toilet very often) or *urgency* (a sudden urge to go to the toilet). People with MS may also have trouble *voiding*, when you can't empty the bladder properly, and this could manifest itself in a number of ways, including incomplete emptying and overflow incontinence. Incomplete emptying is when the bladder does not fully empty, resulting in a considerable amount of urine being left in the bladder (about 100ml or more), and people with this problem often have recurrent urinary tract infections. Overflow incontinence is where the bladder is permanently full and you constantly leak urine. These are all discussed fully in Chapter 4.

People with MS often experience some degree of bowel problem. You may not feel the need to empty your bowel, resulting in a build up of faeces and a leak from your bowel. Or you might have constipation or be unable to fully control the muscles responsible for holding on to faeces.

Diabetes

The body uses glucose (a form of sugar) as fuel. The pancreas produces a hormone called insulin, which helps the body use the glucose properly. Diabetes occurs when the amount of glucose in the blood is too high because there is too little, or ineffective, insulin being produced by the pancreas.

If you cannot produce insulin you are classed as having Type 1 diabetes. If you cannot produce enough, or it does not work properly, you are classed as having Type 2 diabetes. Type 2 diabetes, or Non-Insulin Dependent Diabetes Mellitus (NIDDM), tends to affect people as they get older.

People with diabetes are particularly susceptible to cystitis (an inflammation of the bladder). Because there is too much glucose in the body it is passed out of the body in the urine. Infections can occur because bacteria thrive in an environment with plenty of glucose.

Other symptoms of diabetes are drinking large quantities of fluid, urinating frequently and bouts of diarrhoea. People with diabetes may also experience loss of bladder or bowel control when asleep. You may also have problems with voiding.

The prostate

John
'I was diagnosed with prostate cancer a few years ago. Fortunately, the diagnosis was made relatively early and I had a radical prostatectomy. The operation itself was an ordeal. I had no idea that I would end up incontinent. It was hinted at but no one directly said it, so it came as quite a shock.

'Four weeks after my operation when I went back to hospital to have my catheter removed, I was chatting to the guy in bed next to me when I wet the bed. The Sister came and talked to me and

gave me advice on where to go for help and also talked about the products that I could use. I had bladder problems for two years. With help I managed them and was quite happy. But, I am pleased to say, my bladder problems have now completely cleared.'

All men have a prostate gland. It surrounds the urethra and produces the fluid that carries the sperm when ejaculation occurs.

Prostate problems can occur as a man gets older, if the prostate starts to grow. These include frequency, urgency, urge incontinence and nocturia (having to get up several times in the night to go to the toilet). All of these are discussed later in the book (see pages 33–40).

An operation called a trans-urethral resection of the prostate (TURP) removes some of the enlarged prostate so that symptoms can be relieved. However, in about 1 per cent of cases, this procedure results in persistent urine leakage.

If you have prostate cancer, you may decide to have an operation to remove the whole prostate, called a radical prostatectomy. However, this can also lead to further bladder problems such as leaking urine when you cough, or even leaking all the time (this is estimated to occur in less than 3 per cent of patients).

Stroke

A stroke occurs when a blood vessel or artery is blocked by a blood clot and blood cannot get through to the brain, or when a blood vessel bursts and blood leaks into the brain.

People who have had a stroke may have problems with bladder control as a result. A stroke damages brain cells, so the processes controlled by the affected part of the brain may no longer work normally, or at all.

Senses, speech and movement can all be affected. Bladder and bowel problems may arise because you cannot get to a toilet in time or cannot communicate to someone that you need to go to the toilet. Also, you may be able to sense the need to go to the toilet, but cannot delay it, so have an accident. You may not even remember how to go to the toilet, so may have to learn all over again.

Constipation may also be a problem for people who have had a stroke. It can be caused by nerve damage, so you no longer feel the need to pass a motion. If you cannot move around, eat or drink as you did before, this can also be a contributing factor.

Alzheimer's disease

Alzheimer's disease is a progressive condition which affects mental capabilities. Dementia is the main symptom of the disease. The ability to reason and learn is affected, as is your memory. Eventually, people with Alzheimer's cannot look after themselves, and need full-time care. It is not yet clear exactly what causes someone to develop Alzheimer's.

In the later stages of Alzheimer's, people with the condition often lose control of their bladder, and then their bowels. People with this disease may not be able to get to the toilet in time or may find it hard to get undressed to go to the toilet. They may forget that they need to go to the toilet, might not experience the need to empty their bladder or bowel, or be unsure about what the 'full' feeling means. They might also forget where the toilet is – occasionally people with Alzheimer's go to the toilet in unusual places. It may help if they are taken to the toilet regularly and that the toilet is well signposted.

Parkinson's disease

Parkinson's disease is a progressive condition that affects the central nervous system. People with the disease usually experience three main symptoms:

- your muscles can become rigid or stiff;
- you may experience tremors in parts of your body; and
- your movements may become slower (known as 'Bradykinesia').

People with Parkinson's may have difficulty getting to the toilet in time, or unfastening their clothing when they get there, resulting in an accident. This is mainly due to muscle rigidity and slowness of movement.

Muscle weakness can occur with Parkinson's and this can affect the sphincter muscles, leading to poor control over bladder and bowel functions.

As Parkinson's affects the central nervous system you may not know when you need to empty your bladder or bowel, or you may be unable to hold in urine or faeces, due to a lack of coordination of the sphincter muscles. You might also have urgency or urge incontinence, due to detrusor muscle overactivity.

People with Parkinson's are also likely to have constipation as the digestion process will be slower. This leads to fewer, harder stools.

Bladder and bowel cancer

Cancer occurs when body cells mutate, multiply and interfere with 'normal' cells.

The common symptoms of bowel cancer are changes in your bowel habit, and bleeding from the back passage. This is often associated with weight loss. There are other problems that can cause these symptoms, however. If you experience any of these symptoms you should go and see your doctor.

People who have bowel cancer may need to have part of the affected bowel removed. A colostomy bag may then be necessary to collect the faeces.

Blood in the urine, urgency, frequency and pain when you pass water can all indicate bladder cancer. These could be caused by another condition, such as a urine infection, but it is important to see your GP if any of these symptoms occur.

If the bladder is removed, you will need to pass urine another way. A urostomy operation is usually the solution here. (Colostomies and urostomies are discussed in Chapters 4 and 5.)

Spinal injury

Robert
'I broke my neck in an accident when I was 23 which left me paralysed from the neck down with no control over my bladder or bowel. Since then I have suffered many embarrassing accidents in front of my friends, family and the general public. Much of the time I was too afraid to venture out. All this changed when my

district nurse suggested I see a continence adviser. She listened to all my difficulties and gave much useful advice. After some trial and error, I found products that were a big help. As a result, I have got my life back.'

The spinal cord acts as a 'messaging service' between the brain and parts of the body. If the spinal cord is damaged (as in those born with spina bifida, for example) this 'service' becomes disrupted and the messages do not reach their destination.

Spinal injuries can also occur as a result of breaking your back. Both bladder and bowel function can be affected if the injury occurs to the nerves that control them. You may have either a 'reflex', or 'acontractile' bladder, depending on the location of the injury:

- *The term 'reflex bladder' refers to a bladder which fills and empties automatically when it reaches a certain level. Any sudden movement can cause urine to leak out, much like stress incontinence.*

- *An acontractile bladder is where the bladder cannot contract to empty. Urine leaks out when the bladder becomes full.*

You might also not know when you need to have a bowel motion, or you might not be able to pass faeces naturally.

Childbirth

Childbirth can result in damage to the pelvic floor muscles (the muscles which provide support for the organs in your abdomen). A damaged pelvic floor can result in stress incontinence, where you leak urine when you cough, laugh, sneeze or exercise. In severe cases, you may leak all the time, although this is uncommon.

The extra weight and hormone changes when you are pregnant can put extra pressure on your pelvic floor. A weak pelvic floor can also result in stress incontinence.

If you have a large baby, or forceps are used to deliver your baby, your anal sphincter muscles (rings of muscle that keep the anus closed so no faeces can leak out) might also be damaged. Damage to these muscles can result in subsequent bowel problems. Treatment is available to correct this damage (see page 87).

Menopause

After the menopause, the levels of the hormone oestrogen in a woman's body drop. Oestrogen helps to keep the pelvic floor strong and tight. As the levels of oestrogen lower, you might find that your pelvic floor weakens, which can lead to stress incontinence (see page 33).

Arthritis

The name 'arthritis' means inflammation of the joints. There are over 100 different kinds of arthritis which can affect a variety of joints, such as those in your hands, feet, knees, etc.

When arthritis is at its worst, you may find it hard to move your joints without pain, and you may feel stiff. However, people with certain types of arthritis can have remissions, where the pain and stiffness decreases.

Some people with arthritis (or Parkinson's disease or multiple sclerosis) may find it hard to control their movements, or move their joints freely. This can sometimes make it difficult to get up out of a chair to go to the toilet, walk to the toilet, or unfasten clothing when they get there. Special clothing and products are available, like elasticated trousers and skirts that can make undressing easier (see page 67 for more information), or for people who need to use a catheter, there are appliances that give a better grip for easier insertion. It may also be useful to have a portable urinal or commode close to hand in case you cannot make it to the toilet in time.

Ahmed
'I have arthritis and find it hard to undress quickly. I had some of my trousers altered and they now have Velcro instead of a zip which I find much easier to open – essential as I sometimes have to get to the toilet fast, with little warning, and undress quickly.'

Other causes

There are many other reasons why you might have a bladder or bowel problem. The cause may never be found, even though the problem might persist. Whatever the cause, whether identified or unknown, this book will help you to manage your problem effectively.

2 Help available

Even though it may not feel like it at the moment, there is plenty of help available to help you improve, cure or manage your bladder or bowel problem.

There are healthcare professionals available who can identify the nature and cause of your problem, prescribe treatments for it and describe the different management options that you have.

These healthcare professionals are specialists in the field of bladder and bowel problems and deal with problems like yours every day, so you needn't feel embarrassed or ashamed.

This chapter will outline the role of each of these healthcare professionals. It will also give you pointers on how to talk effectively to your healthcare professional, and tell you what you should expect from them.

The healthcare professionals listed here can be seen privately if you choose. However, for the purpose of this book, we assume that you will see these healthcare professionals under the National Health Service.

Who can help?

The healthcare professionals you will see about your bladder or bowel problem might include:

- GP
- Practice nurse
- District nurse (called community nurse in some areas)
- Continence adviser/continence nurse specialist
- Specialist physiotherapist
- Urologist

- Geriatrician
- Gastroenterologist
- Gynaecologist
- Uro-gynaecologist

Doctors, nurses, some continence specialist nurses and some physiotherapists are members of the primary care team. This means that they are normally the people you will see first about your bladder or bowel problem. If they cannot help you, they will refer you to a member of the secondary care team (such as urologists, uro-gynaecologists and gastroenterologists).

GP/Practice nurse

Your GP or practice nurse might well be the first healthcare professional you see about your bladder or bowel problem. They can advise you about your problem and prescribe medication or suggest other forms of treatment (such as pelvic floor exercises). If the doctor or nurse cannot deal with the problem themselves, and thinks you would benefit most from other sources of help, they can refer you on to another healthcare professional (such as a specialist physiotherapist).

District nurse/community nurse

A district/community nurse carries out 'home visits' to patients who need non-urgent medical care but cannot attend their doctors' surgery or health clinic frequently. They might visit your home, or care home, to change dressings, administer medication or check your blood pressure, for example.

Continence adviser/continence nurse specialist

Continence advisers (or continence nurse specialists) are nurses who are trained in all aspects of bladder and bowel problems. You can telephone some continence services (sometimes called 'continence advisory services') and make an appointment to see a continence adviser yourself. For other continence services, you will need to be referred by another healthcare professional to get an appointment.

If you can ring up and make an appointment yourself (this is called 'open referral' or 'self referral'), it might be best to make your continence adviser the first port of call. *Incontact* (see address on page 102) can give you the number of your nearest continence adviser.

Continence advisers will assess you and recommend treatment or management options. They might recommend medication, or teach you to do pelvic floor exercises, or bladder retraining. Some may also prescribe pads or put you in touch with someone else (usually a district/community nurse) who can prescribe them for you.

Cameron
'I had no idea that there were specialist nurses available. My doctor had never been particularly helpful and it was only when searching the Internet that I realised how many people have these problems. It was a relief to know I wasn't the only one! I got in touch with my continence adviser and she was extremely helpful. I still have problems, but I now know how to deal with them more effectively.'

Specialist physiotherapist

Your physiotherapist will advise you about pelvic floor exercises and the other treatments available. Like continence advisers, you can sometimes make an appointment to see a physiotherapist yourself. For other physiotherapists, you will need to be referred by another healthcare professional to get an appointment.

Urologist

Urologists deal with bladder problems. They can undertake tests to find out what is causing your bladder problem, carry out checks on the prostate, and do biopsies (a small sample of tissue is taken from the affected area and sent for examination).

Geriatrician

Geriatricians specialise in the care of older people. They are experts in conditions primarily affecting older people, such as Alzheimer's disease and arthritis.

Gastroenterologist

Gastroenterologists deal with problems of the digestive system, which can be the cause of some bowel problems. The gastroenterologist will perform tests to identify your problem, its cause, and tell you what treatment options you have. Gastroenterologists do not perform operations, but if they feel that you do need surgery, they will refer you to a colorectal surgeon.

Gynaecologist

A gynaecologist specialises in the female reproductive system. You might need to see one regarding a bladder problem, such as stress incontinence possibly brought on by the menopause. They will assess you and recommend treatment (pelvic floor exercises, bladder retraining, surgery, etc). They may perform operations such as tension-free vaginal tape (TVT) or colpo-suspension (see pages 53–54).

Remember that it is your choice whether or not you have surgery, and remember to ask lots of questions and weigh up the pros and cons (see 'Talking to your healthcare professional' on page 22).

Uro-gynaecologist

A uro-gynaecologist specialises in women's bladder problems. You might go and see a uro-gynaecologist if you are considering having an operation for stress incontinence (see page 33) or a prolapse (see page 39) for example.

What should you expect?

The Department of Health sets national targets, standards of care and guidelines for the NHS. Primary Care Trusts (PCTs) are responsible for planning services and for agreeing contracts with GPs, hospitals, voluntary and private sector providers to ensure that both national targets and local needs are met. Every PCT and NHS Trust has a Patient Advice and Liaison Service (PALS) which gives information about local services and tries to resolve any immediate problems. NHS services are inspected and regulated by the independent Healthcare Commission, which reports regularly on the performance of each NHS organisation.

The guidelines that relate to continence care in the NHS include:

- Good Practice in Continence Services (2000); and

- National Service Framework for Older People (2001).

Good Practice in Continence Services was a result of a working party, formed in 1998, to advise on how to improve continence services. The working party included healthcare professionals and members from organisations that help people with bladder and bowel problems.

The document states: 'The group concluded that organising continence services in an integrated way that focuses on identifying patients, assessing their condition and putting appropriate treatment in place is essential. This guidance sets out a model of good practice to help achieve more responsive, equitable and effective continence services to benefit patients. It aims to:

- raise awareness of professionals to the problems of continence;

- provide practical guidance for the NHS on the organisation of continence services across primary, acute and tertiary care;

- provide advice on the individual assessment and treatment of continence by primary care and community staff; and

- describe targets that can be developed locally.'

The *National Service Framework for Older People* was the result of 'extensive consultation with older people, their carers and the leading professionals involved in the care of older people' and promised 'improvements in health and social care services for older people across the country'.

The National Service Framework recognised the effect that bladder and bowel problems can have on older people: '...continence services are particularly important for older people...Incontinence is distressing for the individual, and for their carers, and is the second most common reason for admission to residential care.'

This document also recognised the need for an integrated continence service and said that this should be in place in all health and social care systems by April 2004.

An integrated service means that you should be assessed, treated and handled in the most effective way possible. If, however, you are unsatisfied with the service you have received, you can contact the Patient

Advice and Liaison Service (PALS) within your local trust. NHS Direct can also advise you and tell you how to contact your PALS – see page 103 for the contact details.

Talking to your healthcare professional

Many people find it hard to speak to someone about their bladder or bowel problem. They often feel embarrassed, or that their problem isn't 'bad enough' to worry the doctor with. Many people tell their doctor about the problem at the end of an appointment for something else.

You must remember that all the healthcare professionals listed above are there to help you. They are used to people speaking about embarrassing topics with them and some of them deal specifically with bladder and bowel problems every day.

It might help if you make a note of any questions you want to ask before your appointment with your healthcare professional. Keep a notebook and pen handy for the week before your appointment and if you think of any questions you want to ask, jot them down. Don't worry if you have a long list. It is important that you fully understand what is happening – it is, after all, *your* body.

Some possible questions your healthcare professional might ask you are:

- How often do you go to the toilet?

- How often do you leak or have an accident?

- When do you have accidents?

- What medicines do you take?

- What do you normally drink?

- How much do you normally drink?

- Is it painful or uncomfortable when you go to the toilet?

- How many times do you get up at night?

If you think they are relevant, jot down the answers to these questions before your appointment.

Take a friend or member of your family with you to your appointment if you would feel more comfortable. Sometimes having someone you know there can help and give you moral support.

If you feel you would benefit from noting down what the healthcare professional says to you during your appointment, take a notebook and pen into the appointment with you. It will save a great deal of worry later on, if you know exactly what the healthcare professional said.

However, if you do feel that you need to ask further questions which you didn't ask at the time, or want to clarify something that was said to you during your appointment, speak to your healthcare professional again. You could also contact NHS Direct, which might be able to help you (contact details on page 103).

It is particularly important to ask questions about any surgery you are planning to have – find out as much about the operation as possible.

Checklist – speaking with your healthcare professional

✓	Don't be embarrassed – healthcare professionals deal with similar conditions all the time.
✓	Note down any questions you want to ask before your appointment.
✓	Take a friend with you if you would feel more comfortable.
✓	Take a notebook and pen with you to your appointment so that you can jot down any important information.
✓	Don't be worried about contacting your healthcare professional again if you want something explained more fully.
✓	Remember that they are there to help you, so be honest and open with them.

3 Dealing with related issues

Bladder and bowel problems can affect you emotionally as well as physically. As they are perceived as embarrassing problems, many people do not like to talk openly about them – they are a taboo subject. People who have these problems sometimes feel that they are the only one in their situation.

This is not true. Millions of people have bladder and bowel problems in the UK alone. More people in the UK have bladder and bowel problems than those with asthma, diabetes and epilepsy put together. But, because asthma, diabetes and epilepsy are more openly discussed, people with these problems know that they are not the only ones with these conditions.

Organisations which help people with these problems are trying to raise awareness of them all the time. Nonetheless, you can feel very isolated if you have a bladder or bowel problem. It is important to look after your emotional side as well as your physical side when dealing with them. This chapter looks at what can be done to help, including coping with stress, how to deal with embarrassing problems, continuing with your sex life, and what to do if you are a victim of discrimination.

How to deal with embarrassing situations

Clare
'People with bladder and bowel problems feel trapped in bodies over which they have no control. They feel mentally, physically and sexually unattractive. This makes you feel an outcast. You build a barrier around yourself. The curse of the problem is not only a physical dysfunction, but also a psychological nightmare.'

Having a bladder or bowel problem can affect your self-esteem, your dignity and your independence. It can also lead to depression and isolation. Many people find it hard to speak to their healthcare professional about their bladder or bowel problem, let alone friends, family or colleagues. Some people live in fear of those people closest to them finding out about their problem. Many people do not leave their homes because they are worried about having an accident.

It is important to remember that you are not alone. It also helps to talk things through with someone else, rather than keep it to yourself.

Siobhan
'My problems affect every aspect of my life. You have to plan ahead and it's hard to socialise freely or to be spontaneous. I miss being able to go out with friends whenever they call. It also affects my marital relationship and sex – fortunately I have a very understanding husband.'

Those who care for you should be understanding, but if you really do feel that you can't speak to them about your problem, and it is getting you down, there are many organisations out there that can help, including the Depression Alliance which provides information, support and understanding and helps with symptoms and treatments (address on page 100).

There are organisations too that can put you in touch with others who have bladder and/or bowel problems. *In*contact (address on page 102) runs a pen-pals scheme, has support groups around the country, and has a website with a chat room and message board. You can share your experiences, exchange advice and tips, and help to support each other.

What to do if you have an accident

So, what do you do if you have an accident? Excuse yourself as soon as possible and get to a bathroom where you can clean yourself up. It always helps to carry a change of clothes, and a few plastic bags with you, in which to store soiled clothes (see the section on 'Travelling with confidence' on pages 67–70).

If someone notices that you have had an accident, be honest with them. You have nothing to be ashamed of. Likewise, if hiding your problem away is affecting your relationships, speak to your friends and family about it. You will probably be surprised at how understanding most people will be.

Sunil

'I have changed my whole outlook on life. I no longer feel ashamed about my problem like I used to, and I am more relaxed about it. Where I used to worry about what people might think, now I think, why worry? It's them who have the problem.'

If you are worried about leaving the house for fear of having an accident, there is an urgency card available, called a 'Just Can't Wait' card. This shows that you have a genuine medical condition that requires urgent use of a toilet. It can be used to jump queues for the toilet, or shown when asking to use a shop's toilets, for example. For your free card, get in touch with *In*contact (address on page 102).

Nathan

'Outings are punctuated with toilet visits. But I refuse to let it rule my life. I'm alright! It's my body that has the 'problems'!'

You may also find it useful to wear dark or patterned clothing. This will help to mask any stains whilst you find somewhere to freshen up and change.

Coping with stress

Eva

'All of you with continence problems know that it's not just the physical side of the issue, but the psychological impact such conditions can have. It is dealing with depression, loss of confidence, loss of self-esteem, and the very real fear of how others will see you. There have been many occasions over the past two years when I have felt worthless as a person, and have been ready to throw in the towel. However, I believe I am more than my disability; I have a great deal to offer and I intend to continue fighting.'

Some problems, like Irritable Bowel Syndrome (IBS), can actually become worse if you are stressed. Worrying about not being able to get to the toilet in time, can make the situation worse, as people who worry often experience more frequent and liquid bowel movements.

The natural methods outlined below are used by some people seeking relief from symptoms brought on, or worsened, by stress. There are many different alternative therapies available. These range from aroma-therapy to reflexology and many more besides. Ask your doctor or continence adviser if they think these treatments might help you – few are available on the NHS.

Acupuncture

Acupuncturists believe that there is a force flowing through our bodies called 'Qi' ('chee'). If the flow of Qi becomes unbalanced, this can lead to health problems. Qi travels along paths called 'Meridians'. By placing needles (which are very fine so you hardly feel them entering the skin) where these Meridians are close to the surface of the skin, the proper flow of Qi can be restored.

Aromatherapy

Aromatherapists use essential oils (from plant extracts) to massage your skin. The aromas from essential oils are believed to have therapeutic properties. Different oils are used for different purposes – some are meant for relaxation, while others work as a stimulant.

Reflexology

Reflexologists believe that each part of the body corresponds to an area on the foot. Your feet are massaged and manipulated to relieve stress or other problems.

Natural remedies

There are natural or herbal remedies available that are said to relieve the symptoms of some bladder and bowel problems. For example, ginger and fennel are said to help digestion problems and cranberry has been proven to reduce the risk of contracting urinary tract infections. (Diabetics should check with their doctor before taking cranberry. Also, people who are taking Warfarin should not drink cranberry juice.) For more information about these natural remedies, get in touch with your nearest herbalist, or visit your local health food shop.

There are many other methods used to reduce stress. Try looking in your local phone directory under alternative or complementary medicines and therapies. The Age Concern publication *Know Your Complementary Therapies* (see page 107) offers further information.

If stress continues to be a problem, or you would rather see a healthcare professional, make an appointment with your doctor who should be able to help.

Sexual activity

Sheila
'My bowel accidents only occur during sex, which is upsetting and embarrassing. Self-image and self-respect are easily destroyed.'

Continuing a sexual relationship when you have a bladder or bowel problem can be a daunting prospect to some people – you may worry about having an accident during sex, for example. The most common piece of advice given to people with any kind of problem with their relationship is to talk to their partner about it.

However, even if you have discussed your feelings with your partner, the practicalities of how to continue a sexual relationship when one, or both of you, has a bladder or bowel problem, can still be a cause for concern. You might be worried about what to do with any devices that you use to manage your problem, like catheters, sheaths or stoma bags.

Here are some things you could try to make continuing your sexual relationship easier:

- Empty your bladder or bowel before sex.

- Men can use a condom to collect any small amount of urine that may be lost during sex.

- Cover the bed with a towel or bedcover with a waterproof backing.

- Catheters can be taped out of the way during sex.

- Light scented candles. Not only are they sensual, but they can also help to mask any odours.

This is by no means an exhaustive list. Speak to your partner to see what ideas you can come up with together. After all, no-one knows your problems and your body as well as you do.

The organisation Outsiders produces a free leaflet about how to avoid leakage during sex, or how to manage the problem if it continues to occur. It also runs a Sex and Disability Helpline (see address on page 103).

If you are finding it hard to discuss your feelings with your partner, and think that seeing a counsellor might help, you could try contacting Relate (address on page 104).

Holidays

Going on holiday can be a concern when you have a bladder or bowel problem. You might be worried about getting to the toilet when on a plane, or be unsure whether you will be able to get supplies of your usual management products when you are away. (See the section on 'Travelling with confidence' on pages 67–70 for some useful information.)

> **Nathan**
> *'It is often overcoming the barriers in our head that is the problem. My advice is get out there and start travelling. Having a bladder or bowel problem does not mean you have to stay at home.'*

Tripscope (see address on page 104) and Holiday Care (see page 102) are organisations that help to arrange hassle free holidays.

If you are concerned about any aspect of your holiday, mention it to the airline, tour operator or hotel management before you go. This will give you time to sort out any queries beforehand and ensure that you can relax and enjoy your holiday when you get there.

*In*contact has a free leaflet about travelling or going on holiday with a bladder or bowel problem (address on page 102).

What to do if you are a victim of discrimination

If you are badly affected by your continence problem, you are covered under the *Disability Discrimination Act*, which came into force in 1995. You have a right to be treated in the same way as people who do not have continence problems. If you are still working, this means that employers can't penalise you for having this problem. You are just as entitled to job offers, promotions, etc that are on offer to people who do not have continence problems.

More information on the Disability Discrimination Act (DDA), including what you should do if you think you are a victim of discrimination, and who is covered under the Act, can be obtained from the Disability Rights Commission (address on page 101).

Money benefits

There are benefits available from the Department of Work and Pensions to people with a disability, and, as we have seen above, you might qualify if you are badly affected by your continence problem. Two of the benefits available from the State are Disability Living Allowance (DLA) and Attendance Allowance (AA).

You might be entitled to the Disability Living Allowance if you find it difficult to get around and/or need help looking after yourself. If you are aged 65 and over and need help looking after yourself, you might be entitled to Attendance Allowance. Further information is provided in Age Concern Factsheet 34 *Attendance Allowance and Disability Living Allowance* (see page 109 for details of how to obtain factsheets).

To see if you qualify for these, or any of the other benefits available, phone the Benefit Enquiry Line for people with disabilities on Freephone 0800 88 22 00. You could also contact the Disability Alliance for more information (details on page 101). Age Concern's annual publication *Your Rights* (see page 107) has more information about all the money benefits that are available to older people.

Support for carers

If you are caring for someone with a bladder or bowel problem, you may be entitled to benefits such as Carer's Allowance. Normally you have to give 35 hours of care each week in order to claim Carer's Allowance. You may also be entitled to help from social services to enable you to take a break. Carers have the right to an assessment of their needs.

Most local authorities have support systems in place for carers. These might include groups where you can meet up with other carers to share experiences and give each other moral support. For more information about carers' rights, or to see if there is a carers' support group locally, contact Carers UK (address on page 100).

4 Bladder problems

There are many different types of bladder problems. They can range from needing to rush to the toilet, wetting the bed or leaking urine when exercising. You may leak a lot or a little. You may only leak at night, or all the time. All can be extremely distressing. It is important to have an understanding of how the bladder works – it may help you to realise the cause of your bladder problem.

With greater understanding, you, together with the advice of your healthcare professional, may be able to reduce, or even cure the problem.

This chapter explains the workings of the bladder and outlines some of the most common bladder problems. It also discusses how to treat and manage bladder problems.

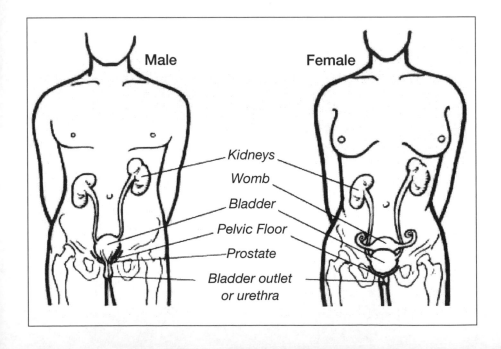

Male

Female

Kidneys

Womb

Bladder

Pelvic Floor

Prostate

Bladder outlet or urethra

How does the bladder work?

Urine passes from the kidneys, down the 'ureters' and is collected and stored in the bladder. The bladder is a muscle, shaped like a balloon. Smooth muscle, called 'detrusor muscle', makes up the outside of the bladder.

In between visits to the toilet the bladder relaxes and fills up. When you go to the toilet the pelvic floor muscles relax, the bladder squeezes, and urine comes out through a tube called the 'urethra'.

There are two other muscles which keep the bladder healthy and prevent any leaks. The 'pelvic floor' is made up of layers of muscles which provide support and hold the bladder in place. Both men and women have a pelvic floor. The other muscle is the 'sphincter', which is a circular muscle that goes around the urethra. The sphincter muscle is normally tight – this seals the urethra so that there are no leaks. When you go to the toilet, the sphincter muscle relaxes so urine can come out.

Types of bladder problems

Some common bladder problems are described below. If you think you have a bladder problem, it is important that you seek the advice of a doctor or continence adviser. The organisations listed at the back of this book can also offer help and advice.

Stress incontinence

Some people leak when they cough, sneeze or laugh. This is called 'stress incontinence' and mainly affects women rather than men. It usually happens because the muscles of the pelvic floor or sphincter are weak or damaged. Stress incontinence is not caused by emotional stress or worry.

In women, these muscles can be weakened during pregnancy by the extra weight and natural hormonal changes. Childbirth can cause more problems; possibly if the second stage of labour is long, the baby is large, or if forceps are used. Some women have some leakage of urine during pregnancy but most bladder problems get better after delivery.

Some women develop stress incontinence after the menopause because the level of oestrogen in their body decreases. This can affect the closing of the urethra, leading to stress incontinence. Even before the menopause, some women may notice that stress incontinence becomes worse before a period.

Occasionally, stress incontinence occurs immediately after having a hysterectomy and some operations on the bladder, although this may only be a temporary side-effect.

People with a bad cough may also be prone to stress incontinence, as repeated coughing puts more pressure on the pelvic floor muscles.

Pelvic floor exercise can help relieve the symptoms of stress incontinence by strengthening the muscles in the pelvic floor. It is important to make sure you are doing the exercises correctly, and that you practice them regularly. (For more information about pelvic floor exercises for women, see page 48.)

Men may also develop stress incontinence after a prostate operation if the urinary sphincter is damaged during surgery. This may be only temporary and can also be helped by pelvic floor exercises for men (see page 48).

Factors that can make symptoms worse for both men and women include:

- smoking – as you may be inclined to develop a cough;
- constipation – as you may strain to pass a motion, which can weaken the pelvic floor muscles; and
- being overweight – as extra body weight puts more pressure on the pelvic floor.

Urgency

You may need to rush to the toilet as soon as you feel the need to go. This sudden urge to go to the toilet is called 'urgency'. People with a 'normal' bladder function can hold on until they reach a toilet, but people with urgency *may* leak if they do not get to a toilet quickly. This is called 'urge incontinence'.

Most cases of urgency are caused by an 'overactive bladder' (see page 36). However, in some people, the cause is never found. You may feel the need to rush to the toilet if you have a 'urinary tract infection' (UTI) (see page 38 for more information).

People with diseases that affect the nerves linked to the bladder, such as multiple sclerosis or Parkinson's, can be prone to urgency/urge incontinence. These kinds of diseases can also impair mobility and prevent people from getting to the toilet in time. This is known as 'functional incontinence'.

'Latch-key' urgency can affect people who already have poor bladder control. This term refers to the need to go to the toilet as soon as you get home and put the key in the door. The knowledge that you will soon be able to go to the toilet, which is often a relief for many people with urgency, may cause your bladder to contract so you have to rush to the toilet. Some people find that hearing running water also has a similar effect.

Bladder retraining, where you teach your bladder to hold on to urine for longer so that you can get to the bathroom in time, can help people with urgency (see pages 50–51 for information about this technique).

Frequency

'Frequency' refers to the number of times you go to the toilet in a day. If you need to go to the toilet very often – more than six times a day – you have 'frequency'.

Frequency can be caused by an overactive bladder (see page 36). The bladder might contract even when it doesn't need to (if your bladder has only a small amount of urine in it, for example). This means you feel the need to go to the toilet more often.

Frequency is often associated with urgency.

Grace
'For many years now I have been too embarrassed to admit that I have a bladder problem. I have always had a tendency to spend a penny a good deal more often than my friends and family. As my husband and I are keen on the outdoors and generally keeping fit, this started to become a real problem for me because you can't always find a toilet when you need one. We also go abroad a lot with my husband's business and the situation can be a lot worse. Recently, the frequency of needing the toilet got so bad that I finally picked up the courage to go and see my continence adviser. She was wonderful, she put me at ease straightaway and told me it was a great shame I hadn't gone for help sooner. I can't

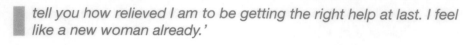 *tell you how relieved I am to be getting the right help at last. I feel like a new woman already.'*

Nocturia

It is 'normal' for some people to get up once a night to go to the toilet, or twice a night if you are older. However, some people have to get up several times during the night. This is called 'nocturia'.

'Nocturnal enuresis' is another name for bedwetting. There are alarms available that can help to wake you up before you wet the bed badly, so you can get to the toilet (see page 64 for more information).

If you have nocturia or nocturnal enuresis, cutting down the amount of liquid you drink before bedtime may help. Also, try not to drink throughout the night – don't keep a glass of water by your bed, for example. However, do make sure that you drink enough fluid throughout the day, as the lining of the bladder can become irritated by urine that is too concentrated.

Both of these problems can be caused by an overactive bladder (see below).

Overactive bladder

Many of the problems mentioned above (urgency, urge incontinence, frequency, nocturia, nocturnal enuresis) are caused by an overactive bladder. These problems are caused when the detrusor muscle squeezes – even when you want to hold on. This is sometimes also called an 'irritable' or 'unstable' bladder. The cause of an overactive bladder is often not known. It can sometimes be caused by an infection in the bladder, or by nerve problems such as stroke, multiple sclerosis or Parkinson's.

An overactive bladder can cause even more problems for people who cannot get to a toilet quickly, such as people with arthritis.

There are several ways to improve an overactive bladder. Bladder retraining, healthy drinking habits, pelvic floor exercises and electrical stimulation may all help: see pages 46–51 for more information. There are medicines that can help too, but these can have side-effects like making the mouth dry and causing constipation (see pages 51–52).

Charles

'My problems, wetting day and night, began at boarding school. The treatment of this condition was for the matron to immerse the 'culprit' in a hot bath into which liberal amounts of disinfectant had been poured. By the age of 10 I had been cured, possibly because of the unpleasant burning sensation I was made to endure.

'So that I should remain aware of my misdemeanours, when others wore their long trousers on Sundays, I was made to wear shorts and required to sleep on a rubber waterproof sheet.

'I remained dry until I had a slight stroke several years ago. Since that time I seem to have lost control of my bladder and on most days and nights I have experienced wetting problems. Thanks to all the help and advice I have received I am able to manage these problems and don't worry that I have to wear protective garments at all times. Once the message gets through that one is far from being alone in having to cope with incontinence, and that help is available, the battle is won.'

Problems in emptying

Sometimes people dribble urine all the time, even without noticing it. Their bladder feels full all the time, and they may need to strain to pass urine. This is called 'overflow incontinence'.

It can be caused by a problem in emptying the bladder. Men, for example, can find it hard to pass urine if they have an enlarged prostate gland.

Some people with overflow incontinence need to go to the toilet very often (frequency).

You may also have trouble passing urine if you have a urethral stricture – a narrowing of the urethra.

Mixed symptoms

It is not unusual to have more than one of these bladder problems at the same time. You may have stress and urge incontinence, or stress and overflow incontinence, for example. This is called 'mixed symptoms'.

Reflex bladder

When you have no feeling that you need to go to the toilet and your bladder empties automatically when it is full, you have a reflex bladder. This usually occurs when there is damage to the nerves in the spinal cord, which interrupts or prevents messages flowing between the brain and the bladder. If there is disruption to these messages, you may not have any idea that your bladder is full.

Going to the toilet at regular intervals can help. You might have to use a catheter, which can be inserted at times throughout the day (an intermittent catheter), or is in place all the time (indwelling or suprapubic catheter). See pages 59–61 for more about catheters.

Urinary tract infection

A urinary tract infection (UTI) is caused by bacterial infection of the bladder wall. The bacteria irritate the bladder lining and you may feel the need to go to the toilet more often and urgently, even if there is only a small amount of urine in the bladder. (It might also be painful and 'burn' when you pass urine.) This is why, if you have urgency or frequency, your healthcare professional will normally rule out a UTI first. There may also be blood in the urine.

A common cause of UTIs is the transfer of bacteria from the anus to the vagina, especially by women wiping from back to front after they have had a bowel movement.

Women are also more at risk of contracting a UTI because they have a shorter urethra. This means bacteria have a shorter journey up the urethra, as well as being closer to the anus than in the male.

'Cystitis' is inflammation of the bladder. It is associated with a painful burning sensation when you go to the toilet. One cause of cystitis is a UTI. Most UTIs can be treated with antibiotics.

'Interstitial cystitis' is also inflammation of the bladder, but the exact cause of interstitial cystitis is unknown. The symptoms of interstitial cystitis can become worse over time. As with UTIs, you may have to rush to the toilet and go more frequently. Interstitial cystitis also causes pain in the lower abdomen.

Bladder stones

Urine contains a lot of waste products from our bodies. Our bodies use the nutrients and other products we need to survive, and then get rid of the rest.

If these waste products which are passed through the kidneys are not dissolved properly in the urine, bladder stones can form. Most people pass tiny crystals of products that haven't completely dissolved, but when these crystals are larger, they can be hard to pass. This can lead to the formation of bladder stones.

Bladder stones can form in the kidney and make their way down to the bladder, or they can form in the bladder itself.

If the stone irritates the bladder, there may be blood in the urine and you may also have difficulty urinating. You may also stop mid-stream if the stone gets lodged in the urethra, although this is very rare.

Stones can be detected by ultrasound or cystoscopy (see page 43 and page 45 for more information about these examinations). If the stones are small, they can be removed during the cystoscopy. If they are larger, you may need an operation to remove them. An alternative method is the use of sound waves to break the stones into smaller pieces so that they can be passed when urinating.

Bladder prolapse

The bladder may drop down and bulge into the vagina. This is known as a 'cystocele'. Women may experience urinary incontinence, a 'dragging' feeling or frequent urinary tract infections due to difficulty in emptying the bladder fully. Frequency, urgency and stress incontinence are also symptoms of bladder prolapse.

Pessaries, which are made of plastic and are normally ring-shaped, can be placed into the vagina to help push the bladder back into the right position. Surgery can also be carried out to repair the prolapse.

Bladder cancer

One of the common symptoms of bladder cancer is blood in the urine. The blood may also clot, causing an obstruction, which can mean that you have trouble urinating. There can be a burning feeling when you go to the toilet and you may need to go more frequently than usual. These symptoms may be caused by some other problems, such as a UTI, but should always be checked out by your doctor.

A cystoscopy, where an instrument called a cystoscope is inserted into the bladder through the urethra, can be carried out to check for bladder tumours (see page 45 for more information).

If the cancer is only present in the lining of the bladder it is called a 'superficial' tumour. This can usually be removed by a probe inserted through a cystoscope. If, however, the cancer has spread to the bladder wall muscle, it is called an 'invasive' tumour. Surgery, chemotherapy and radiation treatment can be used to treat an invasive tumour.

Prostate cancer

Some men with prostate cancer have no symptoms at all. Others may find it difficult to pass urine and have blood in it when they do. There may also be low back pain and weight loss. Some men find out that they have cancer of the prostate when they go in for surgery to reduce an enlarged prostate.

When you have prostate cancer, the texture of the gland may become firmer. This is felt when your doctor carries out a digital rectal examination (this involves the doctor inserting one finger into the back passage to feel the texture of the prostate gland through the lining of the bowel).

Prostate cancer can spread to other parts of the body. Those most commonly affected are the lungs, the bones and the lymph nodes.

If the cancer has not spread to other areas of the body when it is discovered, a radical prostatectomy can be performed. This is an operation to remove the entire prostate.

Other treatments for prostate cancer include:

• brachytherapy (where radioactive seeds are implanted into the prostate);

• cytoreduction (an injection of drugs that block testosterone and shrink prostate cancer); and

• cryosurgery (which freezes cancer cells).

Tests for bladder problems

After visiting your doctor or continence adviser, they may think it necessary to carry out some tests to find out more about your bladder problem and how it can be managed, treated, or, in some cases, cured.

Try not to worry about the tests. Your healthcare professional will have performed these tests many times with many different people. (See page 22 for advice on talking to your healthcare professional.)

Some of the more common tests used for identifying and investigating bladder problems are described below. Your doctor or continence adviser will be able to give you more information about any of the tests that they think are necessary.

Pad test

To see how much urine you leak over a period of time, a pad test might be carried out. One method involves you drinking around 500ml of water and then, after about 30 minutes, a pre-weighed incontinence pad will be placed in your underwear.

You will then be asked to carry out some gentle exercises for about an hour. After this, the pad will be removed and weighed again. This will show how much urine you have leaked whilst performing the exercises.

You may also be asked to collect all the pads you wear at home for a day or two. All these pads will be weighed together to see how much urine you have leaked during the day(s).

Internal examination

The doctor or continence adviser will insert their fingers inside the vagina (for women) or back passage (for men). They will then ask you to try and squeeze their fingers with your pelvic floor muscles. This will show them how strong your pelvic floor muscles are. For men, this test can also be used to see if the prostate gland is enlarged.

Mid-stream urine test

A mid-stream urine (MSU) test is carried out to check for infections. Infections can cause a lot of bladder problems, so it is important that these are ruled out first.

You will be asked to start urinating into the toilet, then hold for a couple of seconds, then continue into a sterilised container. A sample taken mid-stream is more representative and won't contain impurities from the skin around the urethra.

Your doctor or continence adviser will only require a small sample, so you can remove the container after a few seconds and finish urinating into the toilet or urinal.

The sample will be sent to a laboratory and checked under the microscope. A sample from the specimen is spread onto a special plate that encourages bacterial growth. In the centre of a plate is a disc, with other discs, impregnated with different antibiotics, around it. The plate is kept in a warm place for several days so that the bacteria can grow and multiply. The plate is then examined to see where growth has occurred, allowing the laboratory expert to see exactly what kind of bacteria are present. This process means that it takes several days to get your result back from the laboratory.

If there is a significant number of bacteria, pus or leucocytes (white blood cells) present, this means that there is an infection. Antibiotics are usually prescribed for UTIs.

You will be asked to return to the doctor or continence adviser after completing your course of antibiotics. You may then have to give another MSU. If this comes back clear, meaning that the infection has been cured, but you are still having bladder problems, further tests may be necessary to determine the cause of your problem.

Andrea
'The continence adviser was really nice and put me at ease straightaway. She talked me through the procedure, explaining exactly what was going to happen to me and what I needed to do. She was friendly, discreet and caring. Once I got talking to her, I almost forgot where I was.'

Residual urine test

If you have trouble emptying your bladder completely, the urine that is left can stagnate and lead to urinary tract infections. Your doctor or continence adviser can check to see if you have any urine left in your bladder after you go to the toilet (called 'residual urine').

There are two ways that this test can be carried out. Your healthcare professional may use an ultrasound machine to take a bladder scan, which measures the amount of urine left in your bladder (see below), or they may insert a catheter (see page 59) into your urethra to drain the urine that is left in your bladder and then remove the catheter. If you are not used to using intermittent catheters, this method can be a little uncomfortable.

Ultrasound

An ultrasound can be used to provide the doctor with a full picture of your bladder. A probe that sends out sound waves is moved over your abdomen and the resulting picture is displayed on a monitor.

Your doctor may ask you to have a drink a short time before the ultrasound so that your bladder is full, which can help them get a clearer picture of how your bladder is working.

Ultrasounds are completely painless. They can detect abnormalities such as obstructions or an enlarged prostate.

Urodynamics

Urodynamic testing measures the way that the bladder contracts to start the flow of urine, and how much pressure there is in the bladder and urethra.

There are three investigations which make up urodynamic testing. These are 'cystometry', 'flow rate' and 'urethral pressure profile'.

Cystometry

You will have a tube made up of two catheters placed in your urethra. One measures bladder pressure and the other is used to fill the bladder with a saline (salt) solution. Another tube will be placed in your rectum or vagina to measure pressure in the abdominal cavity. The two catheters that measure pressures in the bladder and in the abdomen are con-nected to a machine that will produce a graph.

Your bladder will be filled via the catheter. You will be asked when you feel the need to go to the toilet. More saline will be inserted into the blad-der until you reach the point where you can comfortably hold the fluid in, but feel as though you would be unable to hold any more. The catheter that is used to fill the bladder with the saline will then be removed. The person carrying out the test will then get you to stand up and cough. Any leaks will be noted. You will then be asked to urinate into a flowmeter, which measures your flow rate.

Flow rate

A flow rate test measures how long it takes to empty your bladder, and whether the flow of urine is even, or if it stops and starts. This test can be used to see if you have any problems that make passing urine difficult.

You will be asked to urinate into a special container that measures the millilitres of urine you pass per second. The results are shown on a graph. If you have no obstructions, the graph will be smooth and curved.

Dorothy
'It really made a difference knowing exactly what to expect and why the test was being done. My continence adviser came with me to the clinic and there was a female clinician doing the test, which I felt helped. I was treated with great sensitivity.'

Urethral pressure profile

This test records the pressure along the urethra as the catheter is with-drawn from the bladder. This can determine how well the urethra is func-tioning.

Ambulatory urodynamics

Technology is available that allows in-depth testing to be carried out over a number of hours, with little disruption to the patient – the patient can even move around whilst they are being monitored.

Cystoscopy

Sometimes your doctor may need to have a look inside your bladder to find the cause of your bladder problem. A cystoscope is a long tube that can be inserted into the urethra. It has a camera attached to its end so that an image can be shown on a monitor.

There are two kinds of cystoscope – a rigid cystoscope or a flexible cystoscope. The rigid cystoscope is usually inserted whilst you are under local or general anaesthetic. The flexible cystoscope can be inserted fairly easily if used with some lubricating gel.

The person carrying out the test can direct the cystoscope easily to reach every part of the bladder.

Bladder cancer can be detected. If the doctor or nurse notices any abnormalities and suspects that you may have cancer, you will probably need a biopsy – although biopsies are carried out for other reasons too. Any biopsy will be sent for examination in a laboratory.

Prostate-specific antigen

Prostate-specific antigen (PSA) is a protein that is produced by the prostate. The level of PSA produced by your prostate can be measured by taking a blood test.

A higher level of PSA may indicate that you have prostate cancer. However, the test is not conclusive and the level of PSA can increase if you have an enlarged prostate which may not be cancerous. Generally, the lower the PSA reading, the less likely you are to have prostate cancer. A higher reading normally indicates a problem, which may or may not be cancer.

Intravenous urogram

This test can be used to trace the urine flow through your urinary tract. A dye is injected into a vein in your arm and you have an x-ray. The dye can be seen on the x-ray moving through your bloodstream, into your kidneys and on into your bladder through your ureters. The doctor will be able to see any irregularities, such as stones, a tumour or an obstruction.

Treatment for bladder problems

Once you have visited your doctor, continence adviser or other health-care professional, and they have diagnosed your problem, they will outline the treatment options available to you.

There are many treatment options available and some will be more effective for some people than others. You will probably need to go back to your healthcare professional for regular check-ups to assess how effective the treatment is.

Treatments range from pelvic floor exercises, to medication, and, as a last resort, surgery. Your healthcare professional should encourage you to think carefully before deciding about having surgery. There are many treatments available without the need for surgery that you might be able to explore beforehand.

As always, you should consult your doctor, continence adviser or other healthcare professional before starting any form of treatment described here.

Healthy drinking habits

It is important to drink enough each day. Try to drink at least six cups or glasses of fluid each day. If you normally drink less than this, then increase the amount you drink gradually.

Your doctor or continence adviser might calculate how much you should drink according to a 'fluid matrix'. A fluid matrix suggests that you should drink according to your body weight – those who weigh more need to drink more, while those who weigh less will need a smaller intake of liquid.

The liquid you drink can affect bladder function. It is best not to drink too much tea, coffee, cola or fizzy drinks containing caffeine as these can irritate the bladder and make your problems worse. (There are alternative decaffeinated products available but if you change over to these, do it gradually – caffeine is addictive and withdrawal symptoms such as headache can occur if sudden withdrawal takes place.) Alcoholic drinks can irritate the bladder too.

Instead, drink plain water, fruit juice, fruit or herbal tea and cordials, but avoid blackcurrant as its skin acts as a 'diuretic' (making you need to go to the toilet more often). If you pay attention to what you drink you will notice which drinks cause problems.

Drinking one or two glasses of cranberry juice every day can help people who often get urine infections, as the cranberry has a property in its skin that helps to coat the bladder, making it difficult for bacteria to stick to it. However, the acids in some fruit juices can make things worse for some people, so always check with your doctor or continence adviser as there are specific conditions and medications, such as Warfarin, where cranberry juice would not be advised.

It may be useful to use a 'bladder diary'. This is a chart that you can use to record how much you drink, how often you go to the toilet and how often you have an accident. An example of a bladder/bowel diary can be found in the Appendix on page 92. Your doctor or continence adviser might ask you to fill one in, or you could make a record for a couple of days before your first appointment. This will give your doctor or continence adviser a clearer idea of your symptoms.

Irene
'I have had urge incontinence for the past five years. By controlling my diet I have had considerable success at managing this problem. I noticed that acidic food like citrus fruits, fruit juices and tomatoes made my problems a lot worse. By cutting out these items the irritation lessened.'

Healthy eating

Eating healthily can help some bladder problems. Of course, the benefits of a healthy diet are not just limited to your bladder either.

If you have a balanced diet, this can help prevent constipation. This is important, because if you are unable to empty the bowel, you may feel the need to strain, which can weaken your pelvic floor.

Being overweight can also make bladder problems worse. Extra weight puts more pressure on the pelvic floor muscles, which can become weak, resulting in stress incontinence (see page 33).

Pelvic floor exercises

Pelvic floor exercises can help relieve symptoms of stress incontinence by strengthening the pelvic floor muscles.

Both men and women can use pelvic floor exercises, but the exercises are slightly different for each. For both men and women, it is important to see your doctor or continence adviser to check that you are doing these exercises correctly. You also need to practice them regularly to make the muscles stronger. Exercising these muscles is like any other kind of exercise – the more you do, the stronger they get. You can do them anywhere, at any time.

For women

Imagine you are trying to stop yourself passing wind. To do this you must squeeze the muscle around the back passage. You should be able to feel the muscle move. This is the back part of the pelvic floor. Now imagine that you are about to pass urine – picture yourself trying to stop the stream of urine. This is the front part of the pelvic floor.

Slowly tighten and pull up the pelvic floor muscles as hard as you can – this is a slow pull-up. Count how many seconds you can hold on for and then relax. Repeat as many times as you can.

Now pull the muscles up quickly and tightly, then relax immediately – these are fast pull-ups. Count how many times you can do this without resting.

For men

To locate the correct muscles, tense as though you are trying to stop urinating mid-stream or passing wind. You will feel your anus tighten. When you have located the muscles, try and tense them for as long as you can. Let go, then repeat this as many times as you can.

Then, tensing the same muscles, do a series of fast exercises. Do as many of these as you can.

Joan

'I have suffered from incontinence since the birth of my first child. Going anywhere, doing anything, was getting very stressful – particularly since I have been a PE teacher and very active all my life. Pelvic floor exercises have helped strengthen the correct muscle group. I have had to work hard at these exercises, but I am so relieved that I can now walk to the shops – I've even joined a local ramblers group. I now have to continue to practice these exercises, but it is worth the effort for the freedom from embarrassment.'

Vaginal cones

Vaginal cones are weights that are inserted into the vagina and held in place by the pelvic floor muscles. The weights usually come in a set, with each cone weighing slightly more than the last.

They can help you practise pelvic floor exercises more effectively as you have to use the correct muscles to prevent the cone from falling out of the vagina.

Your doctor or continence adviser will be able to advise you about which weight you should start with. When you feel that you can keep the cone in place easily, they might suggest that you move onto the next cone in the set.

Vaginal cones provide a good method of assessing how well the pelvic floor exercises are working. When you move from one cone to the next, you will see that your pelvic floor muscles are getting stronger.

Electrical stimulation

Some people can be helped by electrical stimulation of the pelvic floor. Both men and women can try this treatment. A probe is placed in the vagina (for women) or back passage (for men). The probe carries an electrical current which can help to exercise and strengthen the pelvic floor muscles. This can be useful for people who find it hard to do pelvic floor exercises in the normal way. Electrical stimulation can also help to improve the overactive bladder and reduce urgency and frequency.

This treatment is normally carried out under the supervision of a specialist, although machines are available for you to treat yourself at home. Your doctor or continence adviser will be able to tell you more about this treatment.

Biofeedback

Biofeedback can help you to discover which muscles to use, when to use them and how hard to contract them to prevent leakage. This can help you have more control over your urethral sphincter muscles and pelvic floor muscles.

A probe is inserted into your vagina (for women) or back passage (for men). The pressure exerted onto the probe when you squeeze your muscles, as though trying to avoid passing water, will be displayed on a computer screen.

Your physiotherapist or specialist nurse will tell you how much harder, and when, you have to squeeze your muscles to provide effective control over your bladder. You will practise using the screen as a guide at first, and then the screen will be hidden from view so that you will have to rely purely on your own feeling.

Gradually, you should gain more co-ordination and control over your sphincter and pelvic floor muscles. The strength of these muscles will also be improved as you are exercising them during your biofeedback program.

Bladder retraining

Many people with urgency (see page 34) will get into the habit of going to the toilet too often to try and make sure that they do not have an accident. This can make the problem of urgency even worse. The bladder gets used to holding less urine and can get smaller, so it becomes even more sensitive or overactive.

Bladder retraining can help improve, or even cure, an overactive bladder. This is a method that helps the bladder hold more urine and become less overactive. Bladder retraining takes time and determination. A cure does not happen overnight, but it can be successful over time.

Keep a diary or record of how often you pass urine for at least three days (see page 92 for an example of a bladder/bowel diary). Gradually increase the time in between visits to the toilet. For example, if you normally go to the toilet every hour, try and hold on a little bit longer.

When you get the urge to pass water, hold on for a bit – this can be just a minute or two to start off with, and you can sit on the toilet to reassure yourself that it doesn't matter if you have to urinate. Try to hold on a little bit longer each time you feel the urge to go. The urge often stops if you hold on when you feel the first urge to go. Try not to think about going to the toilet – distract yourself by doing something.

Bladder retraining slowly stretches the bladder muscle. As it becomes used to holding more urine, the problems of overactive bladder and urgency can be reduced.

Some people find bladder retraining easy and can do it quickly. Others find it harder and it can take longer. Often it will get easier to overcome the urge to pass water. One day you may realise that you have forgotten all about the toilet for several hours.

Keeping a chart or record throughout training will help you to see the progress you are making.

It is important to drink enough liquid for bladder retraining to work (see 'Healthy drinking habits' on page 46). Some medicines can help reduce the urge to go when you are doing bladder retraining – ask your doctor or continence adviser for more details.

Medication

You should always speak to your doctor or continence adviser before taking any medicine. Some medicines may not be suitable for you, even if they are successful for other people. Never take medicines that are meant for someone else.

Ongoing research means that new medicines are being developed all the time. For example, the first medication for treating stress incontinence has now been developed. It is called Yentreve and its generic name is Duloxetine. Ask your doctor or continence adviser for more information about this medication.

There is also a wide range of medicines available for the treatment of overactive bladder and urge incontinence. The information below is meant as a guide only – it is essential that you talk to your doctor or continence adviser before taking any medicines, listed here or otherwise.

Most of the medicines listed here are antimuscarinic, which help to control overactivity in the bladder by blocking nerve impulses. They can help to treat an overactive bladder and are usually best combined with a bladder retraining programme.

All medicines can have unwanted side-effects. The most common side-effects are also listed here. Please note, however, that you are very unlikely to have all of these, and if you start with a low dose, symptoms are rare.

Drug name	Generic name	Main side-effects
Desmospray	*Desmopressin*	Not recommended for people over 65, those with high blood pressure or MS
Desmotabs	*Desmopressin*	Not for people over 65, with high blood pressure or MS. Can cause headache, stomach pain and nausea
Detrunorm	*Propiverine*	Dry mouth, blurred vision, drowsiness, tiredness
Detrusitol	*Tolterodine*	Dry mouth, constipation, abdominal pain, vomiting, dry skin
Detrusitol XL*	*Tolterodine*	Dry mouth, constipation, abdominal pain, vomiting
Ditropan	*Oxybutynin*	Dry mouth, nausea, constipation, blurred vision, dizziness
Lyrinel XL*	*Oxybutynin*	Dry mouth, nausea, constipation, dizziness
Regurin	*Trospium chloride*	Dry mouth, nausea, constipation, abdominal pain

(*XL stands for extended release – for example 'Detrusitol XL' is released into the body over a longer period than 'Detrusitol'.)

> **Dianne**
> *'I had two urodynamic tests which concluded I had an overactive bladder. I was given an antimuscarinic which helped greatly with discomfort and pain, and regulated how many times I had to go to the toilet.'*

Injectables

Injections of substances which 'bulk-up' the area around the urethra can improve the function of the urethral sphincter in some women, helping those with stress incontinence.

A number of substances are used for these injections, some with better results than others. Fat from the woman herself can be used. This reduces the risk of infection, but the results aren't long-lasting.

The injections can also be carried out using collagen which comes from the cartilage of cattle. This substance is longer lasting than fat. There are many other substances (such as silicone) available, all with varying effectiveness.

The procedure itself takes about 20 minutes and can be done under a local anaesthetic. There are no incisions and most women can go home the same day. Most women, however, have to go for top-ups because the injections are not permanent and effectiveness is lessened over time.

Botox injections used to reduce wrinkles can also be used to treat people with bladder problems. Botox is injected into the bladder wall and can help those with an overactive bladder. (This is a different type of treatment to that of the injections outlined above – Botox does not 'bulk up' the sphincter, but stops the bladder itself from contracting so often.)

Your healthcare professional can run through the different substances available and help you to decide whether this method is right for you.

Surgery

Whatever your particular condition, it is important to really think through the pros and cons of having surgery. Ask your doctor as many questions as you want, and never be afraid to go back or telephone to get more information or a clearer explanation.

Colpo-suspension

A common operation to treat stress incontinence is called a colpo-suspension. This is a major operation that requires a general anaesthetic. The abdomen is opened and the bladder neck is stitched to a nearby ligament. This lifts up the bladder neck and helps to stop leaks from it.

There are two versions of the operation. Open colpo-suspension involves making a large cut in the abdomen. Laproscopic colpo-suspension involves making a smaller cut to do the operation – sometimes called 'keyhole surgery'.

This operation can cause extra problems, such as:

• problems with emptying the bladder (some people need to use catheters after the operation);

• irritable bladder and urgency; or

• pain during sexual intercourse.

Tension-free vaginal tape

Tension-free vaginal tape (TVT) is a relatively new operation for women with stress incontinence. It is usually not suitable for those with neurological disease, for women who have not had their menopause yet or who are considering further children, or for women with other conditions like a cystocele or vaginal prolapse.

The operation is gaining popularity because of its relative simplicity and cost-effectiveness. The procedure can be done as day surgery, with only a local anaesthetic. Recovery time after the operation is less than some operations for this problem. However, it should still not be considered a minor procedure.

The tape is inserted through two vaginal incisions. It runs between the vagina and the urethra, lifting the middle of the urethra. This support can reduce the effect of sudden abdominal stress – the cause of stress incontinence.

There can be problems associated with this operation:

• bleeding;

• bladder injury;

• difficulty emptying the bladder;

• urgency;

• urinary infection;

• tape erosion; or

• damage to the bowel or local blood vessels.

The operation is still fairly new, so long-term success rates and side-effects are not known.

As with all treatments, this operation has its advantages and its risks. Everyone needs to discuss with their doctor the options available to them and the pros and cons of each.

Clam cystoplasty

This is a major operation. It involves cutting open the bladder – like a clam – and sewing a patch of intestine between the two halves. The patch can be made of small intestine (ileocystoplasty) or large intestine (sigmoid cystoplasty). The aim of all of these is to increase bladder capacity and reduce its overactivity.

The operation normally takes 1 to 2 hours. A catheter is put in place during the operation. This is left in place for 7 to 10 days to keep the bladder empty while it heals.

The average time needed in hospital after the operation is 10 days, but complete recovery can take three to four months.

The operation can cause extra problems, including:

- The need to use a catheter – mucus from the patch of intestine can block the bladder outlet. As well as this, the enlarged bladder cannot contract strongly enough to push out all the urine. So most people who have this operation have to use catheters to go to the toilet. This will be for the rest of your life.

- Diarrhoea – since some of the bowel is cut out, diarrhoea and other bowel or nutritional problems can be caused.

- Infections in the bladder – bacteria from the patch of bowel can cause recurrent infections in the bladder and urinary tract.

- *Bladder stones – this operation makes it more likely that people will develop bladder stones. Regular check-ups will make sure that these are spotted at an early stage.*

Heather

'The only remedy was to have an operation to enlarge my bladder and, after some discussion, the doctor suggested I have a clam cystoplasty. All the details and possible results were explained. I was happy to go ahead – I had nothing to lose but everything to gain. The operation went well and I was out of hospital in five days instead of ten. The urologist was very pleased and I see him once a year for a check-up. I now have to self catheterise four times a day because of retention, but I still have a better quality of life.

'Whatever the form, incontinence has a profound effect upon the life of the sufferer and their family. There are many prejudices and taboos associated with this delicate and sensitive subject. It is not socially acceptable to talk about it, but I have come out of the closet.'

Detrusor myectomy

This is a major operation. Also known as an 'autoaugmentation', it involves removing part or all of the outer muscle layer that surrounds the bladder. It aims to reduce the amount and strength of bladder contractions of an overactive bladder.

The operation normally takes 1 to 2 hours. A catheter is put in place during the operation. This is left in for 7 to 10 days to keep the bladder empty while it heals.

The average time needed in hospital after the operation is 10 days, but complete recovery can take 3 to 4 months.

The operation can cause extra problems, including the need to use a catheter. Since the muscle has been removed, the bladder cannot contract strongly enough to push out all the urine. So many people who have this operation have to use catheters to go to the toilet.

Urostomy

For some bladder problems your healthcare professional might suggest a urostomy. These problems might include bladder cancer, or a problem with the bladder's function where bypassing it is the only option. It is an operation that involves bringing the ureters out of your abdomen, thereby bypassing the bladder completely. A piece of the bowel is used to join the ureters to the abdomen. The hole that is made where this new tube comes out is called a 'stoma'.

A bag, called a urostomy bag, will be fixed to the skin around the stoma with an adhesive. This will be used to collect the urine and can be emptied at regular intervals. There are also night drainage bags available that are larger, so you don't have to get up during the night to empty them (see page 61 for more about drainage bags).

Cystectomy

This is an operation to remove the bladder. This may be necessary if you have bladder cancer that cannot be cured using chemotherapy, for example. The ureter will be brought out through a stoma (see above).

Lucile
'Anyone considering any kind of surgery should get as much information as possible from their doctor. You can't try before you buy, but you can make a carefully calculated decision.'

Managing your bladder problem

If your bladder problem hasn't been completely cured by the treatments outlined here, there is a vast range of products which can help.

It is worth experimenting, not only with different types of product, but with different makes of the same product. This will help to ensure that you choose the right product.

Remember that your continence adviser will be able to suggest appropriate products. PromoCon, an organisation that gives information on the products available for people with bladder and bowel problems, will also be able to answer your queries (see page 103 for contact details). You can also contact your nearest Disabled Living Centre which will be able to advice you (national address on page 101).

Pads and pants

There are two main types of pads and pants: disposable and reusable. Disposable pads and pants are worn once and then thrown away. Reusable pads and pants can be washed and used again and again.

Disposable pads and pants
There are many different shapes and sizes of pads and it is important that the correct type and size is used. Some are suitable for small leaks, while others are useful for people who have more severe problems.

Some pads can be worn in your normal pants. Other pads come with their own pants to hold them in position or need special pants to keep them in place. There are three main types of pad:

- **Pads without waterproof backing** should be used with special waterproof pants. The pad is inserted into a pouch which holds it in place. There is generally a 'stay-dry' fabric between the pad and your skin – this lets the urine go into the pad, but should stop it feeling wet against your skin. This type of pad is used for light or moderate leaks of urine.

- **Shaped pads with a waterproof backing** can be inserted into your own pants, or held in place by special net underpants, or pants with a special pouch in them. These pads generally have a 'stay-dry' layer which goes next to the skin and a waterproof plastic backing to stop urine leaking out of the pad. This type of pad is used for all levels of leakage.

- **All-in-one shaped pads** are sometimes more suitable for bigger leaks. These pads are designed like children's nappies, with adhesive tapes which fix at the sides to hold the pad in place. These pads usually offer good protection, provided they fit well. There is a waterproof backing material all around the pad which offers protection against leaks. All-in-one pads can be worn without underwear. They should only be used when shaped pads have failed to manage the leakage problem – they can cause skin problems as the skin does not get an opportunity to breathe properly.

Washable pads and pants

Washable pads are available in many different styles and sizes. Washable products can be more comfortable and over time they can be a cheaper option than disposables.

Washable pads are not easy to wash by hand, so a washing machine is usually necessary. They can be slow to dry too, so it is useful to have some spare ones.

Pants with built-in absorbent pads are popular. There are Y-front styles for boys and men, and ordinary knicker styles for girls and women. These are really only suitable for light incontinence or dribbles.

Pull-on 'trainer' pants are made of very absorbent material on the inside, with a waterproof outer layer and elasticated waist and legs to keep them secure and to stop leaks.

Some people prefer towelling nappies, used with plastic pants, especially for night-time protection. These can be more comfortable than disposable pads.

After wetting a pad, get to a toilet to change the pad as soon as possible. Good hygiene is essential to prevent odour and avoid skin problems. (Skincare and odour control are discussed on page 66). Soiled pads or clothing should be put into an airtight container or sealed bag until they can be washed or disposed of. Do *not* flush disposable pads down the toilet.

Always consider using the most discrete product to manage the leakage, rather than the largest one 'just in case'. This may help you to feel less conscious of your problem or anxious that others may see it through your clothes.

Catheters

A catheter is a thin tube. It is used to drain urine from the bladder. Catheters are useful for people who cannot empty the bladder properly.

There are two kinds of catheter: intermittent or indwelling. Intermittent catheters are used at times throughout the day. Indwelling catheters stay in place all the time. The type of catheter you need will depend on the type of problem you have.

Intermittent catheters

These are inserted at intervals throughout the day, or when you feel the need to go to the toilet. Once the urine has drained out, the catheter is removed. This is called intermittent self-catheterisation (ISC). Most catheters for ISC are used once and then thrown away. Some are designed to be cleaned and reused.

There are three main types:

- **Plain catheters** are made of plastic and have to be used with a special lubricant before insertion.

- **Coated catheters** have a hydrophilic coating – this means that the catheter is soaked in water for a short while before use and the water makes the coating slippery so that the catheter is easy to insert.

- **Pre-lubricated catheters** are plain catheters which come packed with lubricant so that they are ready to use.

Follow the manufacturer's guidelines when storing catheters.

Many people find it easy to self-catheterise. You need to have good control of your hands because it can be a fiddle (there are special devices available to help you if you find it hard to handle a catheter) and you should have reasonable eyesight so that you can see what you are doing.

If the packaging is damaged, do not use the catheter. It is very important to wash your hands and genitals before touching or inserting the catheter. Once you have washed your hands, do not touch anything else except your catheter.

Hold the catheter by the drainage end and gently push the other end into your urethra. If you are a woman and find it hard to locate your urethra, try using a mirror to see where your urine comes out. You can do it over the bath if it's easier.

To remove the catheter, withdraw it gently and slowly. Don't worry if it doesn't come out first time. Try again, continuing to pull gently.

> **Tracey**
> *'I started using catheters when I was 36 and at first I did feel weird about it, believing I was the only person who had to do this. However, this is not the case – you are not alone.'*

Catheters designed to be used more than once should be cleaned after each use with soap and water, dried with a clean tissue and kept in a sealed plastic bag or container.

Remember to speak to your doctor or continence adviser before using catheters.

Indwelling catheters

An indwelling catheter stays in place for longer periods of time. There are two kinds of indwelling catheters: urethral and supra pubic. A urethral catheter is inserted into the bladder through the urethra. A supra pubic catheter is inserted into the bladder through a hole in the abdomen, a few inches below the tummy button.

You might need to have an indwelling catheter temporarily, after an operation, for example, or for the rest of your life.

Your healthcare professional will insert either a urethral or supra pubic catheter for you. If you have a supra pubic catheter, this will require a minor operation. A urethral catheter is inserted without the need for an operation. Once inserted, indwelling catheters are held in place by inflating a small balloon at the tip of the catheter in the bladder with sterile water.

Indwelling catheters will need changing from time to time (around 4 to 12 week intervals). Your healthcare professional can change the catheter in your home, or in their surgery or urology department. You, or a member of your family, may also be taught how to change it at home. You must not try to remove your catheter without medical advice.

You have two choices when it comes to draining the urine from your bladder. You can use a catheter valve. If you use a valve, urine will be stored in your bladder and you can empty it through the catheter straight into a toilet. Or, you can let the urine flow freely, through the catheter and into a drainage bag (see below).

When the urine flows straight through the catheter into a drainage bag, your bladder will shrink as it gets used to not storing as much urine. For this reason your continence adviser might recommend that you clamp the catheter for some time during the day. This will help to keep a level of urine in your bladder and prevent shrinkage.

Catheters for men are longer than catheters for women. Because of the location and shorter length of the urethra, women with a urethral catheter are generally more susceptible to urinary tract infections (UTIs) as bacteria from the anus can be passed easily up the urethra with the insertion of the catheter. Men and people with supra pubic catheters are still at risk of UTIs, however. It is therefore important to drink lots of fluids (see page 46) which can help prevent UTIs. Good hygiene is also essential – keep the area around the catheter clean.

Incontact (see page 102 for contact details) produces a set of factsheets about catheters.

Drainage bags

Drainage bags collect urine from a catheter or penile sheath. Normally there is a short tube which connects the catheter or sheath to the drainage bag.

There are two kinds of drainage bags: leg bags and night bags. Leg bags are strapped to your leg under your clothes, held in place by straps or a holster. A night drainage bag is much larger and is attached to the leg bag to hold all the urine that drains from the bladder overnight. It can be hooked onto a stand by the side of your bed and it's a good idea to place a basin under the night drainage bag in case of leakage. Drainage bags have a tap at the bottom to let out the urine.

There are different sized drainage bags. Unless you are told otherwise, you should not use a drainage bag for more than one week without changing it. Before you throw the drainage bag away, empty it in the toilet, wash it out and wrap it in newspaper or a plastic bag. You can then throw it in the dustbin.

There is a new product available now called the 'belly bag'. It is worn round the abdomen and is changed every four weeks.

Sheaths

A penile sheath is a sleeve made of latex or soft plastic. The sheath fits over the penis like a condom and is attached by a tube to a drainage bag (see above). Sheaths can be used during the day or at night. Some men prefer them to wearing pads.

It is important to use the correct size of sheath and to put it on properly. The sheath needs to be big enough to allow natural movement of the penis, but not too loose that it might leak or fall off. Most sheath manufacturers provide a kit so you can choose the right size – ask your continence adviser or nurse if you need help with this.

Some sheaths are self-adhesive, while others need a separate adhesive or adhesive strip. Some are fitted each time using an applicator – these may be easier to use if your fingers are not very nimble, although many people prefer sheaths without applicators.

It is important to wash the penis and area around it before putting on a fresh sheath. Keep pubic hair trimmed so that it doesn't stop the sheath sticking properly. Make sure you follow the instructions that come with the sheath when preparing to put it on.

Some people can be allergic to latex. Keep a check that the skin is not becoming red or irritated. Talk to your doctor or nurse if you are having problems with your sheath.

> **Paul**
> *'I have bladder and bowel problems because I have paraplegia (paralysis of the lower limbs). I intermittently self-catheterise, backed up with a sheath and leg bag. As a result I rarely have an accident. I have a routine of manually emptying the bowel each morning. This is very important.'*

Body-worn urinals

Body-worn urinals may be worth considering if penile sheaths are not suitable.

They should be fitted by a specialist – a good fit is crucial for comfort and to avoid leakage. It is also important that you understand how to use the device. The specialist will check that you have sufficient use of your hands to use the urinal, or that you have a carer who can do it.

There are four types of body-worn urinals:

- **Drip urinals** These are designed to contain a moderate amount of leakage. They come with a waist strap with a reservoir or drip bag, which fits over the penis. There is a tap to drain the reservoir. You can connect another drainage bag onto some kinds of reservoirs so you don't have to empty them so often.

- **Diaphragm urinals** These have a flexible diaphragm held in place by straps. The penis passes through the diaphragm into the urinal.

- **Pubic pressure urinals** These are designed for men who find sheaths unsuitable. The urinal is held close to the body by waist and groin straps and the pressure allows the penis to protrude into the urinal.

- **Penis and scrotum urinals** These are designed to contain the whole genitalia. These types of body-worn urinals can also be used by men with a retracted penis (where all or part of the penis withdraws into the body).

Normally two urinals are needed, as you will need to change your urinal during the day. Each urinal should last about six months. After changing your urinal, it should be washed in warm soapy water, rinsed and dried thoroughly. Follow the manufacturer's washing instructions as each product is different.

You should also wash your penis and the surrounding area in the morning and evening. Do not use talcum powder or cream as these can irritate the skin and affect the material that the urinal is made from.

Some urinals are made of latex and some people are allergic to this. If you do have any problems, see your doctor or nurse.

Hand-held urinals

If you need to get to a toilet quickly, you might find a portable urinal useful. Hand-held urinals are particularly helpful when toilet facilities are not close at hand or easy to use.

They can also be of help to carers when lifting is a problem, as it is possible to use them in bed, sitting down or standing up. There are different types available for these different methods of use.

Some urinals are made of lightweight plastic; these are helpful for people who find it hard to hold heavy objects. Some urinals also have a rubber sleeve around the handle to give extra grip. Some have an extra long handle and others are designed so that urine can't spill out. Others come with an absorbent gel that turns urine into a solid to prevent spills.

Some urinals can be folded up and carried in a pocket or bag. This can be particularly useful if you suddenly get caught short in public. Some of these can only be used once, so the cost can add up if you need to use them regularly. Others can be cleaned and reused.

Using a urinal may not be easy at first, but it will become easier with practice. You might like to use an absorbent bed or chair pad in case any urine spills out.

Alarms

If you wet the bed, it might be worthwhile experimenting with an enuresis alarm. These alarms can wake you up when they detect moisture, so you can go to the bathroom and empty your bladder.

Some alarms have a bed pad that is placed under your bed sheets. This sensor pad is connected to an alarm and the alarm sounds, or vibrates when urine reaches it. Other alarms have small urine sensors that can be fitted to underwear and a small alarm that fits to your nightshirt or pyjama top.

Alarms can help you to recognise the feeling that you have a full bladder and to wake up before you wet the bed. Even if this doesn't work and you continue to wet the bed, the alarms should wake you before you get completely damp.

Bed and chair protection

There is a wide range of covers and pads to protect bedding and furniture. There are covers for mattresses, pillows, blankets, duvets, sleeping bags and all sorts of cushions.

Plastic or PVC is the cheapest and most common material used for covers. But plastic covers don't last very long. Plastic becomes hard and then cracks and splits, especially if it is washed often. Plastic can be hot, sweaty and uncomfortable to lie on. So plastic may be best used in the short term – if you are going on holiday or staying away from home for the night, for example.

There are several newer fabrics which contain polyurethane and polyester. These last longer, make less noise and are often more comfortable to use. But they are often more expensive than plastic products. Some materials claim to be anti-bacteriological, which should reduce the risk of smells. Others are described as 'breathable', which may lessen the problems of sweating.

Always check the size of the cushions or mattress you want to protect. Mattress covers are available in all standard sizes, but can bo made to measure too. If you are a restless sleeper, choose a style which fits right round the mattress as it will be less likely to slip off.

A cheaper PVC mattress cover may be enough if you only use it once in a while. For regular use, it is worth buying a fabric that will last longer and be more comfortable. Some mattress covers also have a terry-towelling surface for added comfort.

To minimise smells and make your bedding protection last longer, always sponge the covers with a dilute solution of mild detergent or disinfectant. If you are using an electric blanket, do check with the manufacturer that the mechanism is completely waterproof.

If a bed or chair pad already has a waterproof backing you may not need any other protection. For extra security you may want to use cushion and mattress covers as well as an absorbent pad. Experiment to find out what works best for you.

Skincare, hygiene and odour control

> **Jamila**
> *'I have to wear a pad every time I go out shopping or socialising, unless I am going to be very near a toilet. I am always worried in case I smell.'*

Many people with bladder problems worry about the smell. Fresh urine should not smell strongly. If it does, it may be because of infection, so see a doctor or nurse.

Urine starts to smell if it is exposed to air, so keep wet clothes and sheets in a sealed bag or container until you can wash them. This should prevent unwanted smells.

Good hygiene is essential to prevent smells and skin irritation. Wash well each day and, if possible, each time a pad is changed. When washing use a mild unscented soap and rinse well. Special skin cleansers are also available. Pat dry with a soft towel and avoid rubbing the skin. A small hairdryer is a good way to dry yourself when at home.

When out and about, you can use moist alcohol-free tissues or baby wipes. You may like to use a simple barrier cream to protect your skin, although some creams may affect the way in which your continence products work, making them less effective and more prone to leakage – seek advice from your continence adviser. Avoid talcum powder and scented washing products. If you find it difficult to wash yourself, ask your nurse to arrange for help.

If the skin becomes red or sore, check if the cause is a pad or other management product that you are using. Ask for help from your doctor or nurse if the skin becomes broken or if pressure sores develop.

Use pads, pants or other products that you find comfortable and that do not leak. You may have to try several types before you find the best one for you. Any leaks or spills should be dealt with as soon as possible. With careful personal hygiene it is often possible to prevent soreness.

Try not to wear tight-fitting clothes. If they are tight, they may rub and cause soreness – loose-fitting clothes will also help the area to breathe.

Easy-off clothing and other aids

If you find it hard to undo your clothing before you go to the toilet, you might find it easier to wear skirts or trousers with elasticated waists, or Velcro instead of fiddly zips and buttons. You can find elasticated waists on skirts and trousers in most clothes shops, but you could also consider having your own clothes adapted. There are organisations that adapt clothes for people with bladder problems. Alternatively, most tailors should be able to alter your clothes – look in your local telephone directory for their contact details. You can also buy clothes with pockets that hold leg bags, or have a flap at the front that can be undone easily when you need to use a urinal, or catheterise, for example. The Disabled Living Foundation will be able to give you more information (address on page 101).

If you find it hard to reach the toilet or use it comfortably, PromoCon (details on page 103) will be able to advise on the range of products available to help – such as raised toilet seats.

Travelling with confidence

Your bladder problem need not stop you from going out, visiting friends or going on holiday. All you need to do is plan ahead. Once everything has been taken care of, you can relax and enjoy your holiday when you get there.

Before you go

If you are looking for help planning your journey, you could contact Tripscope, which offers an information and advice service (details on page 104). Holiday Care also provides information about transport, accommodation and attractions in the UK and overseas (details on page 102).

Take an adequate supply of all the products you use – pads, pants, catheters, sheaths, drainage bags, wet wipes and flannels. Order the extra supplies you need for your trip in plenty of time.

If you are travelling in the UK or Ireland, it might be possible to post a package of your supplies ahead. This will save on luggage space. Tell your holiday accommodation to expect a package and ask them to store it for you until you arrive.

If you think you might change the way you manage your problem for the trip (like switching from intermittent catheters to an indwelling catheter), try it out at home first. If there are any problems, you can sort them out before you go. Remember to consult your continence adviser before changing the way you manage your problem.

There might not always be adequate toilet facilities available when travelling. If you use an intermittent catheter, you might like to change the type you use to one that requires minimal handling, or is self-lubricating. (See pages 59–61 for more information about catheters.) PromoCon can advise you on the range of catheters available. *In*contact also has a set of factsheets about catheters.

It is not necessary to tell your holiday accommodation that you have a bladder (or bowel) problem before you go. But, even if you don't tell them, you will feel more relaxed if you have a chat with the accommodation staff before you go. You can ask them about laundry, disposal and washing facilities. If you intend to do your own laundry, a few coat hangers, a portable washing line and pegs will help.

It is a good idea to take a bag containing your 'clean-up kit' wherever you go. This should contain all the supplies you need (pads, wet wipes, plastic bags, etc). You could also take a change of clothes and a toilet roll with you.

Janice

'I carry a large shoulder bag with me wherever I go that has everything I might need if I have an accident: a change of clothes, plastic bags so I can throw wet pads away, or store wet clothes in until I get home, wet wipes and a small mirror so I can see what has gone wrong. It's a lifesaver.'

Check with your airline or coach company before you go to see if you can have extra luggage allowance, if need be. You might need a letter from your doctor confirming that you have a medical problem and outlining the products and medications that you use. This letter can also be useful when going through any security checks.

The journey

If you are unlikely to have easy access to a toilet, you might want to use a more absorbent pad than usual for the trip. A chair pad can give extra confidence and comfort when sitting for long periods.

If you contact your airline, train company or coach operator before you go, you might be able to book a seat near the toilet.

If you use an indwelling catheter, make sure you take at least one spare with you. Ask your nurse to help you practice changing them. If you use drainage bags, you might want a larger capacity bag for the journey.

Drink plenty of still water when flying to avoid the risk of dehydration.

Loose-fitting clothes are more comfortable when travelling. If you wear a skirt or trousers with an elasticated waist, going to the toilet and changing will be easier.

When you arrive

A change in temperature when on holiday can affect your bladder (and bowel) habits. In hot weather, for example, you can easily dehydrate, so you should drink more water. If you are concerned about the quality of tap water, buy bottled water.

Changes in the food you eat can lead to constipation and diarrhoea, so be careful when choosing meals.

When you are on holiday it is important to look after your skin as you may find that you are in a wet pad for longer than usual if you are stuck on a plane, coach or somewhere with no toilets. (See 'Skincare and hygiene and odour control' on page 66.)

If no toilets are available, a 'Just Can't Wait' card can help (available from *In*contact). You can show this card when asking to use the toilet of a shop, restaurant or other business. It doesn't guarantee you access to their toilet, but it proves you have a medical condition which requires the urgent use of a toilet. Even if they don't let you use their toilet, they might be able to point you in the direction of the nearest public facilities.

You might also find it useful to apply for a RADAR (The Royal Association for Disability and Rehabilitation) key. For a small fee, you will be sent a key giving you access to disabled toilets throughout the UK which use the National Key Scheme (see page 104 for RADAR's contact details).

Roger
'My advice to anyone with a bladder or bowel problem is to get out there and start enjoying life. It's easy to convince yourself that you can't go on holiday, or travel into town. But how will you know you can't unless you try?'

Travelling checklist

If possible, post some supplies ahead. This will save on luggage space.

Contact your airline to see if you can have extra luggage allowance.

Ask your doctor if they can provide you with a letter outlining the products and medication that you use.

If you are considering changing the way you manage your problem when you go away, try it out at home first.

If flying, remember to take extra supplies in your hand luggage to allow for delays.

Wear loose-fitting clothes for the journey – they are more comfortable.

If you are worried about the quality of tap water on holiday, buy bottled water.

Take a small bag full of the things you need to clean-up: wet wipes, change of clothes, pads, plastic bags, handwash, etc.

Get a 'Just Can't Wait' card. This is useful when no public toilets are available – *In*contact can send you one.

If you would like more advice about travelling with a bladder problem, *In*contact (address on page 102) produces a free booklet called *Travelling with Confidence*.

5 Bowel problems

There are many different types of bowel problems. They can range from needing to rush to the toilet, not being able to go, or pain when you do. You may leak a lot or a little. You may only leak at night, or all the time. All can be extremely distressing.

It is important to have an understanding of how the bowel works – it may help you to realise the cause of your bowel problem. With greater understanding, you, together with the advice of your healthcare professional, may be able to reduce, or even cure, the problem.

This chapter explains the workings of the bowel and outlines some of the most common bowel problems. It describes some of the more common tests for identifying and investigating bowel problems. It also discusses the treatment options as well as products which can help with management of problems.

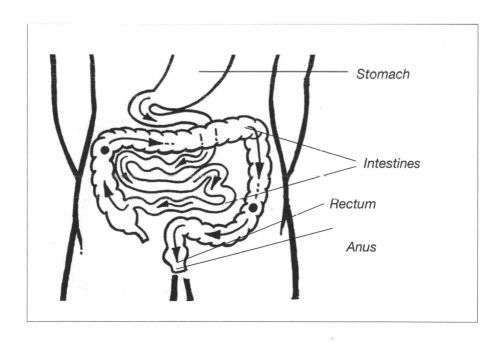

Stomach

Intestines

Rectum

Anus

How does the bowel work?

The bowel is a long tube that carries food from the stomach to the 'rectum'. As the food travels along the bowel, it is digested. Useful nutrients are absorbed along the first part of the bowel (small intestine). Waste that is left at the end of the journey is called 'faeces' or 'stool'.

This waste matter travels from the small intestine to the large intestine (the 'colon') and on to the 'rectum', where it leaves the body through the 'back passage'. The back passage consists of the anal canal and the anus (the hole where the faeces come out).

Different people have different bowel habits. Most people who have a bowel movement more than three times a week and pass good textured faeces (not too hard or too soft) can be said to have 'normal' bowel behaviour.

Some common bowel problems are described below. If you think you have a bowel problem, it is important that you seek the advice of a doctor or continence adviser. The organisations listed at the back of this book can also offer help and advice.

Types of bowel problems

Some common bowel problems are described below. If you think that you have a bowel problem, it is important that you seek the advice of a doctor or continence adviser. The organisations listed at the back of this book can also offer help and advice.

Diarrhoea

A common problem is diarrhoea. This is when faeces are loose and watery. Diarrhoea can cause some people to have frequent and urgent desires to go to the toilet. Sometimes they cannot reach a toilet in time and there is a leak. There are many causes of diarrhoea, including:

- an upset tummy;
- infection or diseases of the bowel;
- some medicines (eg antibiotics);
- eating too much fibre;
- using too many laxatives; or
- anxiety and stress.

Constipation

People who have bowel movements less than three times a week may have constipation. Faeces can become hard inside the bowel so that they are difficult to push out. Constipation can be caused by:

- not eating enough fibre or roughage;

- not drinking enough;

- lack of exercise;

- ignoring the fact that you want to go to the toilet;

- some medicines (eg some painkillers); or

- some neurological diseases, such as Parkinson's disease, which can slow down the digestive process.

If you find it hard to have a bowel movement, do not try to push harder. Straining can cause other problems like haemorrhoids (piles). Straining may also lead to sphincter damage (see page 74).

Flatulence

Flatulence (or wind) can be caused by many things. Experimenting with different foods and drinks can help reduce flatulence, as some foods can produce more gas than others. Try avoiding beans, cabbage, nuts and spicy foods. Tea, coffee and fizzy drinks can also give you wind.

People with diverticular disease (see page 76) can also be prone to wind. Faeces can become trapped in pockets in the colon and gasses can build up. This may lead to excess wind and pain.

> **Davinda**
> *'I suffer from terrible wind. It can be so embarrassing. But I can control it by avoiding certain foods like beans and curries. I've also stopped drinking cola and drink water and fruit squash instead.'*

Haemorrhoids

Haemorrhoids, also known as 'piles', are swollen veins in the back passage. The veins can become swollen when there is increased pressure to the back passage. This can occur if you strain when you are constipated, for example. Haemorrhoids are also common in people who are pregnant, as more pressure is placed on your back passage.

The most common symptoms are bleeding when you go to the toilet, itching and pain around the back passage.

There are creams and suppositories available for the treatment of haemorrhoids. If they persist, you can have surgery to remove them.

Damage to the sphincter muscles

The anus is surrounded by two rings of muscle, one external and one internal, that make up the anal sphincter. The sphincter normally keeps the anus closed, so no faeces leak out. You do not have to think about controlling the internal ring of muscle. The external ring of muscle, however, can be used as a 'back-up' that you control if you need to hold on. You can feel this muscle working if you squeeze, as though you are trying to hold in wind.

If you damage your external sphincter muscle, it may not be possible to hold on until you get to a toilet. This is called 'urge faecal incontinence'.

If you damage your internal sphincter muscle, faeces may leak out after you empty the bowels or if you sneeze, cough, or lift something heavy. In more severe cases, faeces can leak out all the time.

The most common cause of sphincter muscle damage is childbirth. The muscles around the anus can stretch or tear. This is more likely to occur if the baby is very large, or if forceps are used.

Some operations, like surgery to remove haemorrhoids, can damage the sphincter muscles. A rectal prolapse (see page 75) can also weaken the sphincter muscles.

Damaged sphincter muscles might be improved by surgery (see page 87 for more information).

Irritable bowel syndrome

The main symptom of irritable bowel syndrome (IBS) is a combination of pain in the abdomen and irregular bowel habits. There may be other signs like feeling bloated, passing runny mucus instead of faeces, constipation, or pain when going to the toilet. You may also need to get to the toilet quickly (urgency).

IBS may be exacerbated by stress and anxiety. In some people, certain foods can act as trigger, so it may be worth experimenting with the type of foods you eat (see 'healthy eating' on page 82). Medicines called antispasmodics can also help by relaxing the muscles in the colon (see page 85).

Nerve damage

If there is damage to the nerves which make the bowel work, faecal leakage can occur.

Conditions such as multiple sclerosis or Parkinson's disease, or a spinal injury, can cause bowel problems by damaging nerves that transmit signals from the brain to the bowel and back again. This may mean that you no longer feel the sensation of needing a bowel movement. People with these conditions may benefit from implementing a 'bowel programme'. This ensures that you put aside time for having a bowel movement, often with the help of a laxative. This can help prevent accidents as the bowel is cleared out regularly.

Rectal prolapse

A rectal prolapse is when the rectum hangs down into the anal canal. If you have a rectal prolapse, you may leak faeces. A rectal prolapse may occur following childbirth, or be exacerbated by straining whilst constipated. In many cases, the reason for the prolapse is unknown.

An operation called a rectal prolapse repair can be carried out to put the rectum back in the proper position. This repair can be carried out through an incision in the abdomen, or through the anus.

If your rectum pushes into the vagina, forming a bump, this is called a rectocele. If you have a rectocele, faeces may become trapped in the pocket formed, making it hard to have a bowel movement. A ring pessary (a ring-shaped plastic device) can help – ask your continence adviser for more information.

Anal fissures

Anal fissures are small splits around the anus. They can open when you have a bowel movement and may continue to hurt for some time afterwards. They may also bleed. The muscles around the anus may also go into spasm which can make the problem even more painful.

You can help to prevent the fissures from reopening by trying to avoid constipation, thereby keeping your faeces smooth and easier to pass. Warm baths can also help to relieve the pain.

Diverticular disease

This is a condition that affects the colon. Small pockets poke through the muscle along the colon. The pockets rarely cause a problem to the person with diverticular disease, unless they become inflamed (this is known as diverticulitis). This can occur when faeces becomes trapped in the pockets. Diarrhoea and constipation can both occur if this happens. In more serious cases, this inflammation can be life-threatening.

It is still unclear what exactly causes diverticular disease and little research has been carried out, but it is a common disease in older people.

Valerie
'I have suffered from diverticulitis for about eight years. Sometimes I don't have a problem for a week or two, but never knowing when I am going to have a bad day makes life miserable at times. I have a flat on a sheltered housing complex. There are many nice trips I could go on, but I am always too frightened to venture far in case I need to go to the toilet quickly.'

A high fibre diet and mild painkillers may help people with diverticular disease. Surgery to remove the affected part of the colon can also be carried out in severe cases, which may result in having a colostomy (see page 86).

Crohn's disease

Crohn's disease can affect any part of the digestive system. The whole of the bowel wall can become inflamed, leading to strictures (narrowings) of the bowel. The bowel may also form adhesions to other parts of the bowel, other organs around the bowel, or the skin around the bowel. This is known as the formation of 'fistulas'.

The symptoms vary depending on what part of the system is affected. However, the main symptoms of Crohn's are diarrhoea, weight loss and abdominal pain or bleeding. A colonoscopy (see page 79) can help diagnose Crohn's.

The disease can go into remission, so you may not notice any problems at all, but then flare up again.

There is no known cure for this disease, but medication can keep it under control. Surgery can also be carried out to remove affected parts of the bowel.

Colitis

Colitis is an inflammation of the lining of the colon or rectum, and sometimes even the eyes, skin and joints. This may lead to ulceration, and as the ulcers heal, the colon or rectum may become narrower due to the resulting scar tissue. 'Proctitis' is the name given for inflammation of the rectum only.

The major symptoms of colitis are diarrhoea containing blood, and the constant urge to go to the toilet even though nothing comes out. You may also have abdominal pain.

Anti-inflammatory medication or steroids can help. Colitis can be cured by surgery in severe cases to remove the colon. This is a major operation which means that either a pouch will be made out of the small intestine (ileo-anal pouch) and connected to the anus so that faeces can be passed in the usual way, or a stoma bag will be needed to collect the faeces (see page 86).

Bowel cancer

Common symptoms of bowel cancer include a change in bowel habits (the number of times you go to the toilet, or the consistency of your faeces), bleeding from your rectum, which can show up in your faeces, and a lump and/or pain in your stomach.

These symptoms may be caused by some other problem, but should always be checked out by your doctor.

Bowel cancer can be genetic. You are more at risk of contracting bowel cancer if an immediate relative had bowel cancer. A high-fat diet, lack of exercise and high alcohol intake or smoking can also contribute to the disease. If you have had ulcerative colitis, you may also have a higher risk of getting bowel cancer.

There are a number of tests that can be carried out to see if you have bowel cancer. These include sigmoidoscopy, barium enema and colonoscopy (more information about these tests is given below).

Screening for bowel cancer can help detect cancer at an early age and may especially benefit those who are more at risk of developing bowel cancer (such as those with a family history of bowel cancer). Screening can be carried out by flexi sigmoidoscopy using a flexible sigmoidscope (see page 79). Another method examines your stool sample for any sign of blood – if blood is present, you would then go on to have a colonoscopy. However, screening for bowel cancer in this way is not yet available on the NHS, but plans are being made to introduce it.

Surgery is often but not always necessary to remove the cancer. The part of the bowel affected by cancer is removed and the two ends joined together. Sometimes it isn't possible to join the two ends and the end of the bowel has to be brought out through the abdomen. This is known as a 'colostomy' or 'ileostomy', depending on the part of the bowel that is affected (colostomy for the large intestine, or colon, and ileostomy for the small intestine, or ileum). A bag will then be used to collect the faeces (see page 86).

Chemotherapy and radiotherapy can be used to prevent the cancer from spreading further along the bowel, or to other organs (known as secondary cancer).

Tests for bowel problems

After visiting your doctor or continence adviser, they may think it necessary to carry out some tests to find out more about your bowel problem and how it can be managed, treated, or, in some cases, cured.

Try not to worry about the tests. Your healthcare professional will have performed these tests many times with many different people. (See page 22 for advice on talking to your healthcare professional.)

Some of the more common tests used for identifying and investigating bowel problems are described below. Your doctor or continence adviser will be able to give you more information about any of the tests that they think are necessary.

Stool specimens

Similar to a urine sample, a specimen of your faeces may be required to find out if any infection, parasite or blood is present.

To collect a stool sample, sit on the toilet and pass the faeces onto a piece of toilet paper. Then, using a disposable spoon, take a spoonful and put that and the spoon into a sterilised container. Remember to wash your hands afterwards. The stool sample will be sent to the laboratory for testing.

Proctoscopy/Sigmoidoscopy

Sometimes your doctor may need to have a look inside a part of your bowol to find the cause of your bowel problem. A proctoscope is a short tube that can be inserted into a part of the bowel (through the anus) and gives the doctor a clear view of the bowel.

There are two kinds of scope – a rigid scope or a flexible scope. The rigid scope might be inserted using local anaesthetic gel. The flexible scope can be inserted fairly easily if used with some lubricating gel.

A proctoscope is used to examine the anus and rectum, and a sigmoid-scope is used to examine the rectum and sigmoid colon.

The doctor can direct the scope easily to get a complete picture of the part of the bowel they are investigating.

Colonoscopy

This test uses a longer scope which can provide a picture of the whole colon, sometimes using a small camera to send pictures to a monitor. The bowel needs to be prepared beforehand (making sure it is completely clean of all faecal matter) which takes 20 to 40 minutes. It may be carried out after a mild sedative has boon administered as it can cause some discomfort.

A colonoscopy can help detect diverticular disease and colon cancer or any other bowel disease.

David
'I was worried about going in for my colonoscopy, but I asked the doctor a lot of questions beforehand and he put my mind at ease.'

Barium enema

This test can be carried out to check for any abnormalities in the colon or rectum, such as strictures (narrowings), obstructions and lumps.

A paste called barium is inserted into your anus whilst you are lying down. You will then be X-rayed. As X-rays do not pass through barium, the colon and rectum will show up very clearly. Once the test is over, you will be able to go to the toilet to clear out the barium. The test can be uncomfortable as it may make you feel like you have a build up of gas.

You will probably need to use laxatives the night before to clear the bowel out, and you won't be able to eat anything until the test has been completed.

Defaecography

Although similar to a barium enema, this test is done when you are sitting up. A smaller amount of barium is inserted into your rectum, and you do not have to clear out your bowel before the test is carried out.

You will be asked to tighten your anal sphincter muscles and then push as though you are going to the toilet. The barium will, therefore, come out during the test.

X-rays will be taken during the test and the doctor will be able to examine these for any problems. The doctor will get a full picture of how your rectum and anus are working.

Anal ultrasound

A probe is inserted into the anus which enables ultrasound pictures to be taken of the sphincter muscles. This allows your health professional to see if there is any damage to these muscles. This test may be a little uncomfortable.

Anorectal physiological studies

These tests assess the muscle and nerve function of the anus and rectum. A probe is inserted into the anus and the muscle function measured when you are at rest and when you try to squeeze. A balloon may also be inserted into the recturm and gently inflated to simulate build up of stool in the rectum, assessing your ability to feel the presence of stool. Sometimes other tests are done using a low-intensity electrical current to assess sensation or the speed of nerve reaction.

Treatments for bowel problems

Once you have visited your doctor, continence adviser, or other health-care professional, and they have diagnosed your problem, they will outline the treatment options available to you.

There are many treatment options available and some will be more effective for some people than others. You will probably need to go back to your healthcare professional for regular check-ups to assess how effective the treatment is.

Treatments range from changing your diet, to medication, and, as a last resort, surgery. Your healthcare professional should encourage you to think carefully before deciding upon having surgery. There are many treatments available without the need for surgery that you might be able to explore beforehand.

As always, you should consult your doctor, continence adviser or other healthcare professional before starting any form of treatment listed here.

Get into a habit

It is important to make time to have a bowel movement. Most people find that having something to eat or drink as soon as they wake up in the morning stimulates the bowel.

Try and put aside time each morning after breakfast to have a bowel movement, ensuring that you won't be disturbed.

By trying to pass a bowel movement at the same time each day, you might soon be able to get into a bowel habit. You will know when you are likely to need to go to the toilet, thus reducing the risk of accidents.

Healthy eating

June
'If I go out for a meal I have to be careful what I eat as it may cause fairly instant pain, which takes some time to get over, or it may cause pain during the night.'

What you eat has an effect on your bowel movements. The foods that affect some people may not affect others, so you might want to experiment with what you eat. Remember that it's not just your bowels that will benefit from a balanced diet.

Some foods can produce more gas than others – so experimenting with food can help if you are concerned about wind. Try avoiding beans, cabbage, nuts and spicy foods. Tea, coffee and fizzy drinks can also give you wind.

A high intake of fibre can help ensure that you have regular bowel movements that are easy to pass. Fibre can be found in foods such as some breakfast cereals, fruit and vegetables, and wholemeal bread.

However, fibre can cause more problems for people who need to get to a toilet quickly. Also, eating more fibre helps most people with diverticular disease, but, likewise, less fibre can help relieve symptoms in other people. There is very little research in this area, so, again, it is a case of experimenting. What works for you may not work for someone else.

Healthy drinking habits

It is important to drink enough water – you should aim for six glasses a day (and see page 46). This will help hydrate the stools and make them easier to pass. Without a sufficient amount of water in your bowels, the faeces may become hard, and this can result in constipation.

Some people find that drinking a lot of caffeine can cause problems. If this is the case for you, try drinking less tea, coffee and fizzy drinks, or change to decaffeinated alternatives. Artificial sugars, which are found in some diet fizzy drinks for example, can also have a laxative effect.

Biofeedback

When there is a build-up of faeces in the rectum, the internal sphincter muscle should relax and you will know that you need to go to the toilet. Most people can control their external sphincter muscle so that no faeces leak out until they reach a toilet.

Sometimes faeces can leak because you are not controlling the sphincter muscle properly. Biofeedback training can help if this is the case. Biofeedback will help you to recognise when you need to squeeze your external sphincter muscle and how hard you need to do it.

Your specialist nurse or physiotherapist will insert special balloons (or a probe that measures electrical signals generated by the muscles) into your anus. The balloons will record the pressure in your anus and sphincter muscles (likewise, the probe will measure the electrical signals generated).

The nurse or physiotherapist will ask you to squeeze your external sphincter muscle. The pressure or electromyography (the result of the recording of the electrical signals) will show you how hard you are squeezing the muscles. Your specialist nurse or physiotherapist will then show you how much harder you need to be squeezing the muscle.

You will be able to see when your internal sphincter muscle relaxes and will be shown when you need to squeeze your external sphincter muscle to prevent a leak.

Gradually, with practice, you should gain more co-ordination and control over your sphincter muscles. If your sphincter muscles are weak, this training can help as you will be exercising them. Additional exercises can help (see below).

> **Remy**
> *'I feel like I have my life back and no longer have to plan trips around toilets. Before, I felt like I couldn't leave the house in case I had an accident – I had an accident a few times and I was so embarrassed. I decided enough was enough and went to see my local continence nurse. The initial embarrassment I felt when talking to her about my problem soon went – it was far less embarrassing than having an accident in a packed high street, anyway.'*

Exercises

Many bowel incontinence problems are caused by weak sphincter muscles. These can be helped by doing special exercises. With regular practice, the exercises could help to build up your muscles. Check with your health professional to see if these exercises will help you.

To locate your sphincter muscle, pretend that you are trying to hold in a bowel movement, or prevent yourself from passing wind. You should feel the muscles around your anus tighten.

You should sit, stand, or lie, in a comfortable position with your legs slightly apart. Now try and squeeze the muscle for as long as you can. Relax in between each squeeze. Try and do this five times.

Next, squeeze the muscle as hard as you can, then relax. Repeat this five times.

Finally, squeeze the muscles quickly, then let go, then squeeze them again, then let go, and so on. Repeat five times.

Keep practising. If you find the exercises are too difficult, try fewer repetitions at first and build them up. Similarly, if they get too easy, try doing more repetitions.

You can do the exercises without anyone knowing about them, so they should be easy to fit into your daily routine.

Remember to check with your healthcare professional before you start these exercises.

Hold it

Worrying about getting to the toilet in time can make the situation worse. People who worry often experience more frequent and liquid bowel movements. So, if you worry about finding a toilet in time, it is more likely that you will have an accident. Simple retraining can help.

Start by getting to a toilet when you feel the urge, then wait for a minute or so before you open your bowels. Gradually increase the amount of time you wait before having a bowel movement. You should soon find it easier to hold on, even when you are not sitting on the toilet.

Medication

There are a number of medicines available to treat bowel problems. Some of them are outlined below. While some may be helpful, others may not work quite so well or may have side-effects. Remember to speak to your healthcare professional before taking any medication. You might be entitled to some of these medicines on prescription.

Antimotility medicines
These help to slow down movement within the intestine. These are effective at controlling diarrhoea, although one of the possible side-effects is constipation.

Antispasmodic medicines
These relax the intestinal muscles and help to slow down bowel movements to relieve diarrhoea. People with IBS, especially, may benefit from these kinds of medicines.

Bulk-forming preparations
These are commonly used to treat constipation. They bulk-up the stool and improve the regularity of bowel movements.

Laxatives
These may also provide relief from constipation. But take care – taking too many could mean you rely on them to empty your bowel, and can cause diarrhoea too.

Suppositories

Suppositories are capsules inserted into the back passage. They are often used to help relieve the symptoms of haemorrhoids (piles) and can also be used as a laxative to empty the bowel if you are constipated.

Enemas

Enemas are fluids inserted into the rectum. They can be used to clear out the bowel.

There are many other medications available. Please consult your doctor or continence adviser for further information.

Injectables

A form of tissue-bulking material can be injected into the internal anal sphincter to improve its function. The procedure only takes a few minutes, and is performed in the hospital or clinic under local or general anaesthetic, with the patient usually being discharged home the same day.

This relatively new treatment may not be ideal for everybody and there are still risks involved. Talk to your doctor or continence adviser for information about this procedure.

Surgery

Whatever your particular condition, it is important to really think through the pros and cons of having surgery. Ask your doctor as many questions as you want, and never be afraid to go back or telephone to get more information or a clearer explanation.

Colostomy

If your colon or rectum is damaged, you may need to have a colostomy. This involves an operation, carried out under general anaesthetic. Any damaged part of the colon is cut away. The top end of the colon is brought out through a hole cut into the abdomen. This hole is called a 'stoma'. The other end of the colon (nearest the anus) can be closed up, or brought out as well.

Faeces will pass through the colon and out through the stoma. A bag connected to the stoma (called a colostomy bag) collects the faeces.

You will normally have to stay in hospital for between 3 and 10 days. There are specialist stoma nurses who can advise you on how best to look after your colostomy.

> **Rachel**
> *'I had a colostomy about a year ago. It has taken me a while to get used to it, but it is better than being incontinent. It doesn't smell and it is easy to take care of – my stoma nurse told me everything I need to know. It makes some funny noises sometimes, but I have started telling people that I have a colostomy. I don't mind them knowing and most people are fine about it.'*

Sphincter repair

If damaged sphincter muscles are the cause of your bowel problems, this operation may help. The sphincter muscle, which is in the form of a ring, is cut and overlapped. This strengthens any weak points along the muscle, by forming a complete ring.

You will need to stay in hospital for about 4 to 5 days. You will be given laxatives after the operation to soften the faeces, making them easier to pass.

Ileostomy

If the whole of your colon has to be removed (if you have severe ulcerative colitis, for example), you will need to have an ileostomy. This is performed in a similar way to the colostomy above, but the end of the ileum, not the colon, is brought out through a hole in the abdomen.

A stoma nurse will be able to advise you with regards to caring for your stoma.

Rectal prolapse repair

This is an operation to repair a prolapsed rectum. An incision is made into the abdomen and the rectum is put back in the correct position and held there by stitches or a sling.

The operation is carried out under general anaesthetic and you will need to stay in hospital for 3 to 5 days.

Haemorrhoidectomy

If your piles persist and cause you a great deal of discomfort or pain, you may decide to have an operation to remove them. This is called a haemorrhoidectomy. A stitch is inserted into each pile to tie it off and then the pile is removed.

Full recovery takes about 6 weeks.

Managing your bowel problem

If your bowel problem hasn't been completely cured by the treatments outlined here, there are many products which can help.

It is worth experimenting, not only with different types of product, but with different makes of the same product. This will help to ensure that you choose the right product.

Remember that your continence adviser will be able to suggest appropriate products. PromoCon, an organisation that gives information on the products available for people with bladder and bowel problems, will also be able to answer your queries (see page 103 for contact details). You can also contact your nearest Disabled Living Centre which will be able to advise you (national address on page 101).

Pads and pants

Disposable pads and pants are available for people with bowel problems. Washable pads and pants are not recommended for faecal leakage, as it can be hard to remove faecal smells and stains from them. Most people find that pads designed for urine leakage are not the correct shape to deal with faecal leakage.

All-in-one shaped pads are suitable for faecal leakage. These pads are designed like children's nappies, with adhesive tapes which fix at the sides to hold the pad in place. These pads usually offer good protection, provided they fit well. There is a waterproof backing material all around the pad which offers some protection against smells.

Some people use a pantyliner and a g-string to cope with minor leaks. The g-string helps to hold the pantyliner in place between the buttocks.

Stuart

'I wear diaper-style pads for my bowel problem. I used to be concerned about smells, and still am, to a certain degree, in hot weather. But I look after my skin and wash regularly and this seems to combat any problems effectively.'

Remember that it is important to speak to your continence adviser who might recommend other treatment and management options for you.

Anal plugs

An anal plug is inserted into the back passage using a finger. The plug then expands to stop any leaks.

It can be kept in place for twelve hours, but needs to be removed before you have a bowel movement. It has a string attached to it for easy removal, similar to a tampon. Anal plugs are available on prescription.

You can't flush anal plugs down the toilet. When you have removed the plug, wrap it in toilet paper and put it in the bin. Anal plugs should only be used in agreement with your GP or continence adviser.

Drainage bags

There are special drainage bags available purely for the containment of faeces. They are called faecal collectors. They fit around the anus and have a tap and clamp at the bottom, for emptying out either liquid or solid stools. They are rarely used (except by bedbound patients for example). They are quite expensive to buy but are available on prescription. Ask your continence adviser for more information.

Bed and chair protection

There is a wide range of covers and pads to protect bedding and furniture (see page 65 for more information).

Skincare and hygiene

Some people with bowel problems experience sore skin around the anus. Faeces contain digestive juices that eat away at the skin, which can cause soreness. Sometimes it is hard to thoroughly clean the area around the anus and constant wiping can cause irritation. The area will often itch and the skin may also be broken.

It is important to look after the skin to limit the amount of soreness and damage. Wash well each day and, if possible, each time you change a pad or have an accident. Use a mild unscented soap and rinse well. Special skin cleansers are also available. You could use a small mirror to check that you have cleaned the area thoroughly. Avoid scented washing products as these could irritate the skin even more. Pat dry with a soft towel and avoid rubbing the skin. A small hairdryer is a good way to dry yourself when you're at home.

When out and about, you can use moist alcohol-free tissues or baby wipes. You might also like to use a barrier cream, which can help to protect the skin. Ask for advice from your doctor or nurse if the skin becomes broken.

Try not to wear tight-fitting clothes. If they are tight, they may rub and cause soreness. Loose-fitting clothes will also help the area to breathe.

Suzanne
'I find wet wipes are the best thing to use when out and about. You can buy them in small, slim packets that fit discreetly into your handbag. I find they leave me feeling fresher than toilet paper. They have also come in very handy when there is no paper at all in public toilets.'

Clothing

You can buy specially adapted clothes. For example, swimsuits are available that hide a colostomy bag. The Disabled Living Foundation will be able to give you more information on the range of clothes available (address on page 101).

If you find it hard to reach the toilet or use it comfortably, PromoCon (details on page 103) will be able to advise on the range of products available to help – such as raised toilet seats.

Travelling with confidence

Your bowel problem need not stop you from going out, visiting friends or going on holiday (see pages 67–70).

More advice about travelling with a bowel problem is available in the booklet *Travelling with Confidence*, which is available free from *In*contact (address on page 102).

Appendix

An example of a bladder/bowel diary

Time	Comment	Drinks
5am	Woke up to go to the toilet	
7.30am	Leaked before I got to the loo	Cup of tea
9.15am	Made it to the loo in time	

Glossary

Accident: any leak – large or small – of urine or faeces.

Acontractile bladder: the bladder cannot contract to empty. Urine leaks out when the bladder becomes full.

Anal plug: a device that is inserted into your anus to prevent leaks.

Anal sphincter muscles: rings of muscle that keep the anus closed so no faeces can leak out.

Anus: faeces leave the body through this opening.

Aromatherapy: the use of essential oils (from plant extracts) to massage your skin.

Autoaugmentation: another name for detrusor myectomy.

Back passage: the anus.

Barium enema: a paste called barium is inserted into your anus and an X-ray is taken. As X-rays do not pass through barium, the colon and rectum will show up clearly.

Biofeedback: a technique to help you locate your pelvic floor muscles and strengthen them correctly.

Biopsy: a medical procedure in which a small sample of tissue is taken from the affected area and sent for examination to find out more about the problem.

Bladder retraining: a method that helps train the bladder to hold more urine and become less sensitive.

Bladder stones: if the waste products passed through the kidneys are not dissolved properly in the urine, bladder stones can form.

Catheter: a hollow tube inserted into the urethra that is used to drain urine from the bladder.

Clam cystoplasty: an operation for overactive bladder. The bladder is cut open – like a clam – and a patch of intestine is sewn between the two halves.

Colitis: an inflammation of the colon.

Colon: a part of the large intestine.

Colonoscopy: a long thin tube with a camera on the end is inserted into your colon. This enables the doctor or nurse to see a complete picture of your colon.

Colostomy: the top end of the colon is brought out through a hole cut into the abdomen and a bag is used to collect the faeces.

Colpo-suspension: an operation to treat stress incontinence. The abdomen is opened and the bladder neck is stitched to a nearby ligament.

Constipation: the inability to pass faeces on a regular basis.

Continence adviser/ continence nurse specialist: a nurse who specialises in all aspects of bladder and bowel problems.

Crohn's disease: a disease that can affect any part of the digestive system. The main symptoms are diarrhoea, weight loss and abdominal pain.

Cystectomy: an operation to remove the bladder.

Cystitis: an inflammation of the bladder, associated with a painful burning sensation when you go to the toilet.

Cystocele: where the bladder drops down (called a prolapse) and bulges into the vagina.

Cystoscope: a long tube that can be inserted into the urethra and has a camera attached to its end so an image can be shown on a monitor.

Detrusor muscle: smooth muscle that makes up the outside of the bladder.

Detrusor myectomy: an operation for an overactive bladder. All or part of the detrusor muscle is removed.

Diarrhoea: faeces that are too loose.

Diuretic: something (like a certain food or drink) that makes you need the toilet more often.

Electrical stimulation: the use of an electric current to activate and help to strengthen the pelvic floor muscles or calm down an overactive bladder.

Faeces: waste matter that comes out of the anus when you empty your bowels.

Flowmeter: a special container that measures the millilitres of urine you pass per second.

Frequency: the number of times you go to the toilet. If you pass urine more than six times a day, you are said to 'have frequency'.

Functional incontinence: where mobility problems prevent you from reaching the toilet in time.

Gastroenterologist: deals with problems of the digestive system, which can be the cause of some bowel problems.

Gynaecologist: specialises in the female reproductive system.

Haemorrhoidectomy: an operation to remove haemorrhoids.

Haemorrhoids: also known as piles. These are swollen blood vessels around the anus.

Hysterectomy: an operation to remove the womb.

IBS (Irritable Bowel Syndrome): combination of pain in the abdomen and irregular bowel habits.

Ileostomy: the end of the ileum is brought out through a hole cut into the abdomen and a bag is used to collect the faeces.

Ileum: the last part of the small intestine. Nutrients from food are absorbed here.

Incontinence: any leak from the bladder or bowel.

Indwelling catheter: a catheter that stays in place for long periods of time.

Intermittent catheter: a catheter which is inserted at intervals throughout the day, or when you feel the need to go to the toilet.

Irritable bladder: another description for an overactive bladder.

Leak: any amount of urine or faeces that comes out when you are not on the toilet.

Leg bag: collects urine flowing from the bladder through a catheter or penile sheath.

Mid-stream urine test (MSU): a sample taken during the middle of your urine stream (after you start urinating, but before you stop urinating).

Nocturia: having to get up several times during the night to go to the toilet.

Nocturnal enuresis: wetting the bed.

Open referral: the process of making an appointment to see a healthcare professional yourself, without being referred on by another healthcare professional.

Overactive bladder: the detrusor muscle squeezes even when you want to hold on, causing problems such as urgency, frequency and nocturia.

Pads and pants: absorbent pads and pants that help to soak up leaks from the bladder or bowel.

Pelvic floor: layers of muscle which support the bladder and bowel and help prevent leaks.

Pelvic floor exercises: exercises to help strengthen the pelvic floor muscles.

Penile sheath: a sheath fits over the penis and urine passes through it. Normally worn with a leg bag.

Pessaries: made of plastic and normally ring-shaped, pessaries are placed into the vagina to help push the bladder or bowel back into the right position.

Physiotherapist: can advise you on pelvic floor exercises and other treatments available.

Piles: the name often used for haemorrhoids.

Prolapse: where an organ (such as the bladder or rectum) falls out of place.

Prostate: a gland that sits at the base of the male bladder and surrounding the first part of the male urethra.

Prostate-specific antigen (PSA): a protein that is produced by the prostate. The level of PSA produced by your prostate can be measured by taking a blood test.

Radical prostatectomy: an operation to remove the entire prostate.

Rectum: the last section of the bowels.

Reflex bladder: a bladder which fills and empties automatically when it reaches a certain level. Any sudden movement can cause urine to leak out, much like stress incontinence.

Reflexology: reflexologists believe that each part of the body corresponds to an area on the foot. Your feet are massaged and manipulated to relieve stress or other problems.

Residual urine: the amount of urine left in the bladder after you have gone to the toilet.

Sigmoid colon: the lowest part of the colon above the rectum.

Stoma bags: collect urine (after a urostomy) or faeces (after a colostomy or ileostomy). They attach to the opening (or 'stoma') and need to be emptied and/or changed regularly.

Stress incontinence: the leakage of urine when you cough, sneeze or laugh.

Stricture: a narrowing – for example, a 'urethral stricture' is a narrowing of the urethra.

Suppositories: medicated capsules which are inserted into the back passage.

Suprapubic catheter: a catheter inserted into the bladder through a hole in the abdomen.

Tension-free vaginal tape (TVT): a special tape is inserted through two vaginal incisions. It runs between the vagina and the urethra, lifting the middle of the urethra. This support can reduce the effect of sudden abdominal stress – the cause of stress incontinence.

TURP (trans-urethral resection of the prostate): an operation to remove some of an enlarged prostate so that symptoms can be relieved.

Ultrasound: a probe that sends out sound waves is moved over your body and the resulting picture is displayed on a monitor. Can be used to give a complete picture of your bladder or anal sphincter muscles.

Unstable bladder: another name for an overactive bladder.

Ureters: tubes leading from the kidneys to the bladder through which urine travels.

Urethra: the tube that carries urine out of the bladder.

Urethral sphincter muscles: the muscles that constrict the urethra to control the flow of urine.

Urinal: a device used to collect urine when you can't get to the toilet in time, or no toilets are available. They can be hand-held or body-worn.

Urinary tract infection (UTI): this is caused by bacterial infection of the bladder wall. This bacteria irritates the bladder lining and you may feel the need to go to the toilet more often and urgently, even if there is only a small amount of urine in the bladder.

Urine: waste fluid that comes out of your bladder.

Urge incontinence: when you feel the need to get to a toilet quickly, but do not make it in time.

Urgency: a sudden urge to go to the toilet.

Urodynamics: a series of tests that measure the flow of urine and how much pressure is in the bladder and urethra.

Urologist: specialist in the field of bladder problems, prostate problems and the sexual organs.

Urostomy: an operation that involves bringing the ureters out of your abdomen, bypassing the bladder completely. A piece of the bowel is used to join the ureters to the abdomen, where a hole is made so the ureters can be brought out.

Vaginal cone: a weight that is inserted into the vagina to help exercise and strengthen the pelvic floor muscles.

Voiding: passing urine.

Further help

Alzheimer's Society
Gordon House
10 Greencoat Place
London SW1P 1PH
Helpline: 0845 300 0336
Website. www.alzheimers.org.uk
*Care and research charity for
people with dementia and their
families and carers.*

Arthritis Care
18 Stephenson Way
London NW1 2HD
Freephone Helpline: 0808 800
4050 (12pm–4pm, Monday to
Friday)
Website: www.arthritiscare.org.uk
*Information and support for
anyone with arthritis.*

ASBAH (Association for Spina Bifida and Hydrocephalus)
42 Park Road
Peterborough PE1 2UQ
Tel: 01733 555988
Website: www.asbah.org
*Provides information to
individuals, families and carers.*

Association for Continence Advice
102a Astra House
Arklow Road
New Cross
London SE14 6EB
Tel: 020 8692 4680
Website: www.aca.uk.com
*Membership organisation
for health and social care
professionals concerned with
continence care.*

Bowel Control website
Website: www.bowelcontrol.org.
uk
*Information and advice for people
with loss of bowel control.*

British Colostomy Association
15 Station Road
Reading RG1 1LG
Helpline: 0800 328 4257
Website: www.bcass.org.uk
*Provides support, reassurance
and information to people who
have had, or are about to have, a
colostomy.*

CancerBACUP
3 Bath Place
Rivington Street
London EC2A 3JR
Helpline: 0808 800 1234
Website: www.cancerbacup.org.
uk
*Advice and support for people
with cancer and their families and
carers.*

CarersUK
20–25 Glasshouse Yard
London EC1A 4JT
Tel: 020 7490 8818
CarersLine: 0808 808 7777
(10am–midday and 2pm–4pm,
Wednesday and Thursday)
Website: www.carersuk.org
*Provides carers, those supporting
them and others, with national
and local information.*

Continence Foundation
307 Hatton Square
16 Baldwins Gardens
London EC1N 7RJ
Helpline: 0845 345 0165
Website: www.continence-
foundation.org.uk
*Has a helpline staffed by nurses
(9.30am–1pm, Monday to Friday)
and produces a range of patient
information leaflets.*

Cystitis and Overactive Bladder Foundation
76 High Street
Stony Stratford
Buckinghamshire MK11 1AH
Tel: 01908 569169
Website: www.cobfoundation.org
*Gives support to people with
interstitial cystitis and overactive
bladder and their families and
friends.*

Depression Alliance
35 Westminster Bridge Road
London SE1 7JB
Tel: 0845 123 2320
Website: www.depressionalliance.
org
*Information about symptoms of,
and treatments for, depression,
plus a network of local groups.*

Diabetes UK
10 Parkway
London NW1 7AA
Careline: 0845 120 2960
Website: www.diabetes.org.uk
*Help and support for people with
diabetes, their families and carers.*

Digestive Disorders
Foundation (changing its name to Core)
PO Box 251
Edgware
Middlesex HA8 6HG
Tel: 020 7486 0341
Website: www.digestivedisorders.org.uk
Funds research into digestive disorders and provides information to those with them.

Disability Alliance
Universal House
88–94 Wentworth Street
London E1 7SA
Tel: 020 7247 8776
Rights Advice Line: 020 7247 8763 (2pm–4pm, Monday and Wednesday)
Website: www.disabilityalliance.org
Provides advice and information regarding social security benefits and other entitlements.

Disability Rights Commission
Freepost MID02164
Stratford upon Avon CV37 9BR
Tel: 08457 622 633
Website: www.drc-gb.org
Independent body established to eliminate discrimination against disabled people and promote equality of opportunity.

Disabled Living Centres Council
Redbank House
4 St Chad's Street
Cheetham
Manchester M8 8QA
Tel: 0870 770 2866
Website: www.dlcc.org.uk
Free and ethical information, via phone or face-to-face in local centres, about products that can increase disabled or older people's choices about how they live.

Disabled Living Foundation
380–384 Harrow Road
London W9 2HU
Helpline: 0845 130 9177 (10am–1pm, Monday to Friday)
Website: www.dlf.org.uk
Information and advice on products and clothing which help with independent living.

Friends of Fashion Services for Disabled People
The Greenfield Centre
Green Lane
Baildon
West Yorkshire BD17 5JS
Tel: 01274 597487
Provides information and advice, made-to-measure clothes and alterations.

Holiday Care
7th Floor
Sunley House
4 Bedford Park
Croydon
Surrey CR0 2AP
Tel: 0845 124 9971
Website: www.holidaycare.org.uk
*Provides information about
transport, accommodation, visitor
attractions, activity holidays and
respite care establishments in the
UK and abroad.*

Hysterectomy Association
60 Redwood House
Charlton Down
Dorchester
Dorset DT2 9UH
Helpline: 0871 781 1141
Website: www.hysterectomy-
association.org.uk
*Information about having a
hysterectomy and its long-term
health implications.*

IBS Network
Northern General Hospital
Sheffield S5 7AU
Tel: 0114 261 1531
Website: www.ibsnetwork.org.uk
*Advice, information and support
for people with irritable bowel
syndrome.*

**Ileostomy and Internal
Pouch Support Group**
Peverill House
1–5 Mill Road
Ballyclare
County Antrim BT39 9DR
Tel: 0800 0184 724
Website: www.the-ia.org.uk
*Helps people who have had an
ileostomy or ileo-anal pouch.*

***In*contact**
United House
North Road
London N7 9DP
Tel: 0870 770 3246
Website: www.incontact.org
*Provides information and support
and a range of publications for
people affected by bladder and
bowel problems and their carers.*

**ITAAL (Is There An Accessible
Loo?)**
10 Stilecroft Gardens
North Wembley HA0 3HE
Website: www.itaal.org.uk
*Works to improve the provision
of accessible toilet facilities for
disabled people and increase
the public understanding and
appreciation of the personal care
needs of disabled people.*

MS Society

372 Edgware Road
London NW2 6ND
Helpline: 0808 800 8000
Website: www.mssociety.org.uk
*Funds research, produces
publications and runs a helpline
for those with multiple sclerosis.*

MS Trust

Spirella Building
Bridge Road
Letchworth Garden City
Hertfordshire SG6 4ET
Tel: 01462 476700
Website: www.mstrust.org.uk
*Provides information for people
with multiple sclerosis and for
health professionals.*

National Association for Colitis and Crohn's Disease (NACC)

4 Beaumont House
Sutton Road
St Albans
Hertfordshire AL1 5HH
Tel: 0845 130 2233
Website: www.nacc.org.uk
*Provides information and support
to people with Crohn's disease
and ulcerative colitis and their
families.*

NHS Direct

Tel: 0845 46 47
Website: www.nhsdirect.nhs.uk
*Has a 24-hour helpline and
website that provide health
information.*

Outsiders

BCM Box Outsiders
London WC1N 3XX
Tel: 020 7354 8291
Sex and Disability Helpline:
0707 499 3527 (11am–7pm,
Monday to Friday)
Website: www.outsiders.org.uk
*For people who feel isolated
because of social and physical
disabilities.*

Parkinson's Disease Society

215 Vauxhall Bridge Road
London SW1V 1EJ
Helpline: 0808 800 0303
Website: www.parkinsons.org.uk
*Support, advice and information
for people with Parkinson's, their
families and carers.*

PromoCon

Redbank House
4 St Chads Street
Cheetham
Manchester M8 8QA
Helpline: 0161 834 2001
(10am–3pm, Monday to Friday)
Website: www.promocon.co.uk
*Provides information on products
and services relating to bladder
and bowel problems.*

RADAR

12 City Forum
250 City Road
London, EC1V 8AF
Tel: 020 7250 3222
Website: www.radar.org.uk
Run by and for disabled people, representing the needs, views and wishes of disabled people. Runs the National Key Scheme.

Relate

To book an appointment call:
0845 130 40 16
Website: www.relate.org.uk
Relationship counselling face-to-face or via phone and website.

Royal College of Nursing Continence Care Forum

c/o RCN
20 Cavendish Square
London W1G 0RN
Tel: 020 7409 3333
Website: www.rcn.org.uk
Shares information and research relating to continence care.

Samaritans

Tel: 08457 90 90 90
Website: www.samaritans.org
Provides confidential emotional support.

Spinal Injuries Association

Acorn House
387–391 Midsummer Boulevard
Milton Keynes MK9 3HP
Tel: 0800 980 0501 (9.30am–1pm and 2pm–4.30pm, Monday to Friday)
Website: www.spinal.co.uk
Support for people with a spinal cord injury, their families and carers. Publishes leaflets about bowel and bladder management.

Stroke Association

240 City Road
London EC1V 2PR
Helpline: 0845 30 33 100
Website: www.stroke.org.uk
Support for people who have had a stroke, their families and carers. Publishes a leaflet about stroke and continence.

Tripscope

The Vassall Centre
Gill Avenue
Bristol BS16 2QQ
Helpline: 08457 585641
Website: www.tripscope.org.uk
Travel advice and transport information for people who are disabled or have problems getting around.

Urostomy Association of Great Britain and Ireland

18 Foxglove Avenue
Uttoxeter
Staffordshire ST14 8UN
Tel: 0870 770 7931
Website: www.uagbi.org
Helps people who are about to have, or have already had, a urostomy.

About *In*contact

*In*contact is a national charity for people with bladder and bowel problems. Formed in 1989 by a group of patients and health professionals, the organisation provides information and support to people affected by these taboo conditions, as well as their carers and the health professionals who look after them.

A central function of *In*contact is to raise awareness amongst the public and health professionals of these common problems, and the range of treatment and management options available. It aims to break down the stigma that still surrounds incontinence. As a consumer-led organisation, *In*contact views the patient's voice as paramount. It works closely with the National Health Service and the voluntary sector to ensure that this voice is heard. *In*contact aims to act as the mouthpiece for the millions of people in the UK affected by incontinence. The management committee includes consumers, informal carers and healthcare professionals.

*In*contact produces a range of user-friendly information materials including leaflets, product information sheets, a magazine full of readers' experiences, features, pen-pals, letters and all the latest news. *In*contact also provides the telephone number of a local continence adviser (a nurse specialising in all aspects of bladder and bowel problems).

*In*contact also coordinates a network of local groups and helplines around the country for people affected by continence problems – talking to someone who 'knows what it is like' is so important for many. *In*contact provides information and advice to health professionals, patients and carers who are thinking about setting up a local group.

For more information and to find out how *In*contact can help you, phone 0870 770 3246, email info@incontact.org, visit www.incontact. org or write to *In*contact at: United House, North Road, London N7 9DP. *In*contact also has regional offices in Wales (0870 770 3247) and Scotland (0870 770 3248).

Registered charity no. 1085095.

About Age Concern

Age Concern is the UK's largest organisation working for and with older people to enable them to make more of life. We are a federation of over 400 independent charities which share the same name, values and standards.

We believe that ageing is a normal part of life, and that later life should be fulfilling, enjoyable and productive. We enable older people by providing services and grants, researching their needs and opinions, influencing government and media, and through other innovative and dynamic projects.

Every day we provide vital services, information and support to thousands of older people of all ages and backgrounds. Age Concern also works with many older people from disadvantaged or marginalised groups, such as those living in rural areas or black and minority ethnic elders.

Age Concern is dependent on donations, covenants and legacies.

Age Concern England
1268 London Road
London SW16 4ER
Tel: 020 8765 7200
Fax: 020 8765 7211
Website:
www.ageconcern.org.uk

Age Concern Scotland
113 Rose Street
Edinburgh EH2 3DT
Tel: 0131 220 3345
Fax: 0131 220 2779
Website:
www.ageconcernscotland.org.uk

Age Concern Cymru
4th Floor
1 Cathedral Road
Cardiff CF11 9SD
Tel: 029 2037 1566
Fax: 029 2039 9562
Website:
www.accymru.org.uk

Age Concern Northern Ireland
3 Lower Crescent
Belfast BT7 1NR
Tel: 028 9024 5729
Fax: 028 9023 5497
Website:
www.ageconcernni.org

Publications from Age Concern Books

Age Concern Books publishes over 65 books, training packs and learning resources aimed at older people, their families, friends and carers, as well as professionals working with and for older people. Publications include:

Know Your Complementary Therapies *Eileen Inge Herzberg*

Written in clear, jargon-free language, this book provides an introduction to complementary therapies, including acupuncture, herbal medicine, aromatherapy, spiritual healing, homeopathy and osteopathy. Uniquely focusing on complementary therapies and older people, the book helps readers to decide which therapies are best suited to their needs, and where to go for help.

£9.99 ISBN 0-86242-309-0

Intimate Relations: Living and Loving in Later Life *Dr Sarah Brewer*

This book answers the questions that many older people have on loving, as well as sexual relations, in later life. There are many ways of sharing a fulfilling and enjoyable love life, and there is no need for age-related health problems to get in the way.

A rewarding sex life is an important part of well-being and a loving relationship – at all stages of adult life. This unique book will be of interest to everyone, whatever their age, health or sexual orientation.

£9.99 ISBN 0-86242-384-8

Your Rights: A Guide to Money Benefits for Older People *Sally West*

A highly acclaimed annual guide to the State benefits available to older people. Contains current information on State Pensions, means-tested benefits and disability benefits, among other matters, and provides advice on how to claim.

For further information please telephone 0870 44 22 120.

Your Taxes and Savings: A Guide for Older People *Paul Lewis*

An annual guide which explains how the tax system affects older people over retirement age, including how to avoid paying more than necessary. The information about savings and investments covers the wide range of opportunities now available.

For further information please telephone 0870 44 22 120.

To order from Age Concern Books

Call our **hotline: 0870 44 22 120** (for orders or a free books catalogue)

Opening hours 9am–7pm Monday to Friday, 10am–5pm Saturday and Sunday

Books can also be ordered from our secure online bookshop: **www.ageconcern.org.uk/shop**

Alternatively, you can write to Age Concern Books, Units 5 and 6 Industrial Estate, Brecon, Powys LD3 8LA. Fax: 0870 8000 100. Please enclose a cheque or money order for the appropriate amount plus p&p made payable to Age Concern England. Credit card orders can be made on the order hotline.

Our **postage and packing** costs are as follows: mainland UK and Northern Ireland: £1.99 for the first book, 75p for each additional book up to a maximum of £7.50. For customers ordering from outside the mainland UK and NI: credit card payment only; please telephone for international postage rates or email sales@ageconcernbooks.co.uk

Bulk order discounts

Age Concern Books is pleased to offer a discount on orders totalling 50 or more copies of the same title. For details, please contact Age Concern Books on 0870 44 22 120.

Customised editions

Age Concern Books is pleased to offer a free 'customisation' service for anyone wishing to purchase 500 or more copies of most titles. This gives you the option to have a unique front cover design featuring your organisation's logo and corporate colours, or adding your logo to the current cover design. You can also insert an additional four pages of text for a small additional fee. Existing clients include many prominent names in British industry, retailing and finance, the trade union movement, educational establishments, private and voluntary sectors, and welfare associations. For full details, please contact Sue Henning, Age Concern Books, Astral House, 1268 London Road, London SW16 4ER. Fax: 020 8765 7211. Email: hennins@ace.org.uk

Information Line/Factsheets subscription

Age Concern produces more than 45 comprehensive factsheets designed to answer many of the questions older people (or those advising them) may have. These include money and benefits, health, community care, leisure and education, and housing. For up to five free factsheets, telephone 0800 00 99 66 (8am–7pm, seven days a week, every week of the year). Alternatively you may prefer to write to Age Concern, FREEPOST (SWB 30375), ASHBURTON, Devon TQ13 7ZZ.

For professionals working with older people, the factsheets are available on an annual subscription service, which includes updates throughout the year. For further details and costs of the subscription, please contact Age Concern at the above Freepost address.

We hope that this publication has been useful to you. If so, we would very much like to hear from you. Alternatively, if you feel that we could add or change anything, then please write and tell us, using the following Freepost address: Age Concern, FREEPOST CN1794, London SW16 4BR.

Index